JOIN THE SELF-CARE REVOLUTION

MODULE TWELVE: CELEBRATE LIFE & PAY IT FORWARD!

HOSTED BY: DR ROBYN BENSON & KEVIN SNOW

Featuring: Janet Mueller; Rev. Adara Walton, N.D., PhD; Marcella Vonn Harting, PhDc; Deborah Koppel Mitchell; Bill Parravano; Charley Johnson; & Marcia Wieder

2014

First Printing: 2015

ISBN: 978-1-312-21927-4

Self-Care Revolution™
2905 Rodeo Park Drive East, Building #3
Santa Fe, NM 87505
505.474.8555

www.jointheselfcarerevolution.com

Disciaimer:

This site/book is not designed to and does not provide medical advice, professional diagnosis, opinion, treatment, or services to you or to any other individual. Through this site and linkages to other sites, Santa Fe Soul, LLC, (SFS) provides general information for educational purposes only. The information provided in this book, or through linkages to other sites, is not a substitute for medical or professional care, and you should not use the information in place of a visit, call consultation or the advice of your physician or other healthcare provider. SFS is not liable or responsible for any advice, course of treatment, diagnosis or any other information, services or product you obtain through this site.

IF YOU BELIEVE YOU HAVE A MEDICAL EMERGENCY, YOU SHOULD IMMEDIATELY CALL 911 OR YOUR PHYSICIAN. If you believe you have any other health problem, or if you have any questions regarding your health or a medical condition, you should promptly consult your physician or other healthcare provider. Never disregard medical or professional advice, or delay seeking it, because of something you read on this site or a linked website. Never rely on information on this website in place of seeking professional medical advice. You should also ask your physician or other healthcare provider to assist you in interpreting any information in this Site or in the linked websites, or in applying the information to your individual case. Health and medical information changes constantly. Therefore the information on this Site or on the linked websites should not be considered current, complete or exhaustive, nor should you rely on such information to recommend a course of treatment for you or any other individual. Reliance on any information provided on this Site or any linked websites is solely at your own risk.

SFS does not recommend or endorse any specific tests, products, procedures, opinions or other information that may be provided on the linked websites. The linked websites may contain text, graphics, images or information that you find offensive (e.g., sexually explicit). SFS, its licensors and its suppliers have no control over and accept no responsibility for such materials.

These statements have not been evaluated by the Food and Drug Administration. The information in this book is not intended to diagnose, treat, cure or prevent any disease.

Table of Contents

The Self-Care Revolution™ Topics

Module 1: Your Thoughts And Food As Medicine

Module 2: Heart And Breath Matters

Module 3: Transmute And Release Trauma

Module 4: Unleash Your Brain Power

Module 5: Earthing, Electro-Sanitizing, And Growing Your Own Garden

Module 6: Power Of Relationships (Self, Others & Money)

Module 7: Exercise As Medicine

Module 8: Empowerment

Module 9: Power Of Community

Module 10: Be Fabulous At Any Age

Module 11: Power Of Gratitude

Module 12: Celebrate Life And Pay It Forward!

WELCOME TO THE SELF-CARE REVOLUTION™!

MODULE TWELVE of TWELVE: CELEBRATE LIFE & PAY IT FORWARD

Pay It Forward is a term for describing the beneficiary of a good deed and repaying it to others instead of to the original benefactor according to Wikipedia. To become a pay it forward champion in every day life is an excellent self-care choice. Not only does your giving support another, but also simple acts of kindness on a daily basis have a positive physiological effect on your body. Research shows that it increases your good mood hormones oxytocin and decreases the overproduction of the stress hormone called cortisol and so much more.

Listen to this module's experts and join with the Self-Care Revolution to strengthen the network that is weaving the support for all who care to improve health and wellness as individuals, families, in our communities and as part of the global community in stewardship of the earth and one another.

What Is The Self-Care Revolution™?

Launched in January 2013, the Self-Care Revolution is the gift to humanity from the Santa Fe Soul Health and Healing Center and its Founder, Dr. Robyn Benson, DOM. Her caring and passionate heart and commitment arises from travel throughout 70 countries and over twenty-two years of practice and extensive trainings. These experiences have given her an overview, an expansive network and an effective creative approach in dealing with the healthcare crisis in America.

The mission of the Self-Care Revolution™ and our Self-Care Coaches™ (true mentors and guides) is to change the face of healthcare through the fundamentally different approach where "It All Starts with You".

The Self-Care Revolution™ evolved in response to a modern world epidemic where diseases such as diabetes, Alzheimer's, obesity, cancer, fatigue, pain, stress, anxiety, and depression are running rampant. Many people have given up on our current disease-management model of healthcare and are seeking alternative, holistic, and more effective means to facilitate healing.

The vision of the Self-Care Revolution™ is to save millions of lives by transforming the way people look at healthcare. The goal is to teach people that "it all starts with you and within you" and that self-care is the solution to the healthcare crisis we are facing. Basically, almost each and every one of us has the power and ability to heal ourselves through informed choices and a healthy lifestyle.

It is our mission to touch one million lives with the purpose of creating a world of people committed to their Self-Care, thus contributing to healthier communities and, in turn, to a healthier planet.

Why Is Self-Care So Effective?

The Self-Care Revolution™ brings world-renowned experts in traditional medicine, alternative healing, integrative medicine, personal growth, spirituality, new cutting-edge technology, and the expertise of the Self-Care Coaches to support the subscribers in all areas of optimal health and "Self-Care."

The Self-Care Revolution™ is a one-of-a-kind educational and empowering interview series with world-renowned leaders who have agreed to hold nothing back and to give you their best transformational work that will move you toward abundant health and happiness NOW.

We are empowering individuals with the necessary skills, knowledge and practical tools to radically change the course of their health and life.

We have interviewed over 100 top experts and continue to add to the interview series each and every module.

The Self-Care Revolution™ movement creates awareness of reversing and preventing disease, and finding the cure from within. Our priorities are:

- Revolutionizing our members' awareness of whole-body wellness—mind, body and spirit—and supporting them as they take action based on the education and resources we provide.

- Educating our members on self healing, enriching their lives and empowering them to effect change in themselves and their environment. Providing our members with the resources and support to effectively live a healthier, happier, sustainably vibrant life enabling them to actualize their own dreams.

Why Should Self-Care Be Important To You?

Did you know that 40% of all bankruptcies in this country are due to unmanageable healthcare costs due to an unforeseen health crisis? How will you prevent this from happening to you or your family?

It's vitally important that you take the time to ask yourself these questions:

- What are you willing to commit to today to ensure your healthy future?

- What Self-Care strategies will you implement each day that will promote your best daily energy and vitality (food, thoughts, exercise)?

- What is the impact you want to make in the world with your optimal, radiant and sustainable health through your commitment to body-mind-spirit Self-Care?

By purchasing this Module (and investing in the other eleven Modules of this series) you have taken an important step toward Self-Care. We invite you take the next step and become a valued member (for free) of the Self-Care Revolution™, a weekly, educational and empowering tele-seminar and so much more.

Don't take this journey alone; invite your friends and family, too.

For more information on any of the membership levels and upcoming events visit: www.JoinTheSelfCareRevolution.com

This is an exciting opportunity to create powerful changes for yourself and collective wellness worldwide. This revolution is raising awareness to a new level of understanding of what is "The True Health Care".

Join us in this call to action to create a world that works for everyone with health and vitality.

With love from Robyn, Kevin and your Self-Care Revolution team, The Best Gift you can give another is a healthy you!

About Santa Fe Soul Health & Healing Center:

Santa Fe Soul Health & Healing Center for holistic and preventative healthcare is the vision of founder and director Robyn Benson, Doctor of Oriental Medicine. We welcome you into this beautiful space to meet our highly experienced health care professionals where you will learn about the benefits of many services such as Acupuncture, Biofeedback, Chiropractic, Therapeutic Massage and IV Therapies, as well as our innovative leading-edge energy technologies.

Santa Fe Soul was built from the ground up in 2004 as a consciously created sacred space for health and healing with the purpose of offering you the best health care. Our community of practitioners will work together with you to compliment any medical treatment you may be undergoing. For more information, feel free to visit us online:

www.SantaFeSoul.com

JOURNAL

CELEBRATE LIFE AND PAY IT FORWARD!

We are in the final month of the 12-month Self-Care Revolution™ series and this is our final journal. Congratulations to you for staying on this journey and committing to your Self-Care to change your life and those around you!

Consider how your daily Self-Care choices have allowed you to feel and look better and to even be more present, passionate and purposeful each day.

Are you ready to make the world a better place by paying it forward?

For many, when we think of the concept of 'Pay It Forward' you might immediately think of Diana Ross's popular song 'Reach out an touch someone's hand" or the movie Pay It Forward that came out in the year 2000 with Kevin Spacey and Helen Hunt. Be sure to see this movie and see how it ignites your Pay It Forward spirit.

Wikipedia says Pay It Forward is a term for describing the beneficiary of a good deed and repaying it to others instead of to the original benefactor. TO become a Pay It Forward champion in every day life is an excellent self-care choice. Not only does your giving support another, but also simple acts of kindness on a daily basis have a positive physiological effect on your body. Research shows that it increases your good mood hormones oxytocin and decreases the overproduction of the stress hormone called cortisol.

The Pay It Forward spirit can be the ultimate antidote to fear, depression, anxiety, if your not connected to a higher purpose, and when you are simply bored or lonely.

Be the reason that someone is happier today, knowing it does not have to cost a penny.

In gratitude,

Robyn and Kevin and the Self-Care Revolution™ team

Let us know how you are doing. *We are here to support you*

Questions:

Write down 31 things you can do in the next 31 days to help another person, or to give back to your friends, family and community.

_____

_____

_____

_____

_____

_____

_____

_____

_____

_____

_____

_____

_____

_____

_____

_____

_____

_____

_____

Based on all the growth you have experienced since month one of the Self-Care Revolution, how do you feel your positive choices have impacted your family, friends, coworkers and others?

_____

_____

_____

_____

_____

Think back to a time that you gave back to someone else as a result of someone doing something nice for you. How did you feel inside?

_____

_____

_____

_____

_____

What ritual can you set for yourself to allow Pay It Forward to be part of your daily life?

_____

_____

_____

_____

_____

Testimonials:

"The Self-Care Revolution™ is brilliant as it speaks to the only solution for the health care crisis we are in. *Take responsibility for your health.*"
Norm Shealy, MD, PhD

"The Self-Care Revolution™ is on the cutting edge of Americans and our global community taking Responsibility for their Health, Wealth and State of Happiness."
Steve Rose (Health and Wealth Advocate)

"The Self-Care Revolution™ is truly phenomenal, and is a revolution and a movement whose time has come. I can't think of a better cause that we each need to awaken to daily in order to do our great work in the world. All I can say is the speakers have been outstanding."
Vince Hughs (Entrepreneur)

"Self-Care is the True Health Care. That says it all! Thank you for taking me on this fabulous journey with you and your incredible speakers. I am a changed woman from the inside out."
Helen Stucky (Historian, Founder of Wellness Weavers)

"Nothing like Rockin' my Self-Care this year. I feel and look better, and my career and prosperity is better than ever. The tools I have learned are priceless. My Self-Care Lifestyle is here to stay. Watch out world!"
Hillary S. (Hautepreneur, Designer)

Pay It Forward:

A big part of the Self-Care Revolution™ is the "*Pay it Forward*" message, so much so that we dedicated one full month to it, with seven speakers. Why not pass this book forward to someone else after you are complete with it, so that Self Care, the True Health Care message, will awaken in every single person on this planet. And ahhhhh, imagine how much more peace, true joy and connection that will bring into our lives.

WITH LOVE FROM YOUR SELF-CARE REVOLUTION SUPPORT TEAM!

JANET MUELLER

JanetIMueller.com | CEO J Mueller Group LLC and Founder of Leadership In Excellence Academy, Coach, Speaker and Author of "*A Champion's Guide To Thriving Beyond Breast Cancer*"

TURN YOUR CHALLENGES INTO GIFTS - PAY IT FORWARD

Robyn: Hello everyone and welcome to month twelve of the Self-Care Revolution™, celebrate life and Pay It Forward is our theme. All the co-creators of the Self-Care Revolution™ thought long and hard about what the last month would be and we clearly knew that after moving through topics like thoughts and food is medicine and exercise is medicine, unleashing your brain power and power of gratitude and empowerment and all these good things, now it's time to Pay It Forward.

My name is Robyn Benson and I'm a Doctor of Oriental Medicine. I am the Founder of Santa Fe Soul Health and Healing Center and I have to say the way I love to Pay It Forward everyday is to help people achieve optimal radiant and sustainable health through all the tools I have to share. I'm here with…

Kevin: Kevin Snow, the co-host of Self-Care Revolution™ and I'm so grateful to be part of this conversation today. I'm an Intuitive Counselor at Santa Fe Soul and what I share with the world is to help people create clarity in their lives. That is my gift.

Robyn: That's beautiful. We are excited, having a few minutes on our own with our wonderful speaker today, Janet Mueller. Welcome.

Janet: Hi everyone, thank you for having me. I'm grateful to be here and excited to be with you today.

Robyn: We love that you're here. I love the theme of today's talk. I'm going to share a little of your background with our audience real quick and then I'll turn it over to you.

Janet is the CEO of J Mueller Group LLC & Founder of Leadership in Excellence Academy. A messenger, business strategist, coach, transformation teacher, speaker, and a published author. Janet is hired for her expertise to speak around the world on transformation, leadership development and servant leadership. As seen on SNN6, ABC 7 My Sun Coast, and daytime NBC. Janet's 20 years of leadership expertise, study of human psychology, and her talent and gift for coaching has helped her to inspire, teach, and transform lives worldwide.

In the corporate world she's successfully led, coached and trained executives and sales teams in both the direct sales and healthcare industry with fortune 500 and 100 companies. Janet partners with organizations and individuals helping them to get the results they want and become who they aspire to be. She is heart driven, an authentic leader who inspires, teaches and gets results! Janet is grateful to God for giving her a passport to more time having survived a near death experience so she can continue to help and make a difference touching and transforming lives all around the world through her speaking, teaching, coaching, seminars and books.

I want to start with the book you've just written, your first book that just came out a month ago.

Janet: Yes, just published with Morgan James Publishing. I'm very excited to have the book out and I think because the message is similar to yours, it's about serving and helping and healing and giving hope to many people, specifically for those who have breast cancer. One in eight women are diagnosed with breast cancer in our lifetime and I believe this book is a gift of hope that can help them to rise up and move beyond adversity, as have the women and myself in the book.

Robyn: What's the title of the book?

Janet: It's A Champions Guide to Thriving Beyond Breast Cancer.

Robyn: That's beautiful.

Kevin: I love the title. What is your definition of Champion? What does that mean to you?

Janet: Great question. As a girl growing up I was a gymnast, something that I was passion about and for those listening, you probably have a sport or athletic of some type that you participated in growing up and I use the metaphor of the gymnast in the book. As we think about the adversity and challenge that we all have in each of our lives, using the metaphor of the gymnast to help us to power through. If you see the walking being the balance beam of how we move through life and how we use that as a metaphor to balance, to take tiny steps to get from one side to the other. I believe we're all messengers and we're here to help each other cross from one side to the other.

A champion and a champion mindset is really about being positive, the positive psychology and having endurance. It's about realizing that we can choose to see all the adversity and challenges we have as gifts and blessings and then sharing those and paying those forward to help other people. Servant leadership is something I'm extremely passionate about and I believe that when we share the gifts we have we can help to heal spirits, heal hearts around the world.

Robyn: I love that. Can you talk to us about where the inspiration for this book came about?

Janet: I actually lost a best friend to breast cancer at 33 years young. She was a young mom with a son and she was diagnosed late stage, so within 12 months of being diagnosed she was gone. We lost her to breast cancer and I felt called to help and inspire other women around the world, I think, to bond through my own adversity in life that empathy and compassion to want to help inspire and give other women hope.

Her story, giving her a voice and helping her, if you will, to live on and be able to use that for good and to Pay It Forward. It took me into the local community and interviewing seven very courageous women and having them share their stories of how they're surviving and thriving as a way to give other women hope. So I'm blessed and grateful for her friendship, because it inspired the book and the book will definitely help other women around the world.

Kevin: You mentioned about healing and its relevance to this champion mindset. Could you expand a little on that concept of how the champion mindset relates to healing?

Janet: Absolutely. I believe that we all have the opportunity to be mindful in how we view our circumstances and our adversity. One piece of that is mindfully being aware of how we think about our circumstances and we know, as I'm sure you've heard, that with neuroscience we can reprogram the neural pathways and start to be an observer of the thoughts that we have and what thoughts we choose to hold onto and let go of.

So from an empowering standpoint I believe that we can all choose mindfully what thoughts we want to hang onto, the positive and negative and that can be helpful in a positive trajectory in place, so that we can focus on being more positive. I think the second piece is critical and that is faith. I'm a big believer that it's not just about positive thinking, but it's about having that deeper trust and intuitive piece where you pay attention to what you feel, hear and see and your faith plays a huge part.

I think meditation is also a big piece. I just came away from Experts Industry Association and we heard all about the TM meditation that Chris Attwood shared with us and all the benefits associated with that for anxiety, reduction, stress reduction, help with lowering blood pressure and depression. So, I think meditation is such a huge piece also.

Robyn: Is that part of your day-to-day practice Janet?

Janet: Yes it is.

Robyn: That's great. Can you clarify a little more about how a champion mindset has helped you in your life?

Janet: Absolutely. I can share some stories with you that I'm sure many of your listeners can relate to as well. I actually experienced a near death experience over 15 years ago, where I was physically attacked, literally on death's door and I remember in that moment praying 'Dear God, please don't let me die.' I believed that in that moment it was going to be lights out and that I was not going to be here. I choose to see that experience, even though it was traumatic, it also is now a blessing because I see from that that I'm able to serve, to help, to heal and show others empathy and compassion to help them heal through the adversity.

That is a mindful decision that I choose to see that as, as something positive rather than something negative. So I think having that champion mindset has helped me. Again, I go to faith, meditation, the positive psychology and it's really about perspective on how we view our circumstances. We talked about gratitude and having daily gratitude is such a huge piece. A lot of people believe that we have to be happy first to then be grateful but in actuality it's the other way around. The practice of being grateful produces more happiness. I think having that gratitude in our lives every single day, finding something to look for to be grateful for is also huge.

Robyn: Janet, can you spotlight some of the women that are in your book and their stories?

Janet: Yes. One of the ladies in the book is Norma. She was diagnosed at stage 4 breast cancer and in a year she not only had been diagnosed but her husband had passed away. She'd been let go from her job. She lost both her mother and father and found herself literally without insurance. I share her story because I look at that and think my goodness, if someone can have that strength, faith, courage and belief that they can move beyond this and rise up, if someone can go through all that in 12 months, that is a shining example that demonstrates that it is possible for more people to heal and rise up.

Robyn: I love that.

Kevin: How has this impacted your clients?

Janet: Getting a positive result is essential. We're hired to get results for people. I know for my clients, I've actually helped students that have seen me go through the process of writing the book, going into the community, serving that level and I've actually been able to help two other clients produce books and get their stories and message out in a very short amount of time. So I love this interview about celebrating life and paying it forward, because to me that's what we're here for. We're here to serve one another and to help each other get those results so we can help more people. I'm excited. I've been blessed and able to help a couple people write their own books and share their messages as well, in a short space of time.

Robyn: I know that's part of the word celebration to, where the Pay It Forward energy comes so powerfully from a place of celebration, of having made it through a major journey as you said earlier, a challenge. How important do you think this courage, creativity and passion are towards happiness?

Janet: I believe that creativity, you know you hear the expression that anxiety is the handmaiden of creativity. I do believe that creativity turned inward can lead to anger and depression. We see one in five women diagnosed with depression and it gets me curious into how are we moving away, especially with the children in schools and as women, by not speaking out, not standing up and sharing our voice and our message. How is that impacting our overall health? I'll go to gratitude here because I actually give lots of gratitude to someone I consider a great mentor, Brendon Burchard, who has helped me rise up, speak out and share my voice as a way to serve and help others.

I do believe that coming out of the corporate world, we are educated away from sharing our ideas and being creative, and not really being allowed to be out of the box, think out of the box and be innovative. I think we have a long way to go in helping people being more creative and encouraging that from a health point of view and certainly in the schools with young girls. I think the more creative we are we can probably tackle some of the diagnoses for depression that I'm curious if they are actually real diagnoses.

We talk a lot about going back to who we were as kids and what it is we love to do. I remember creating math textbooks in my dad's garage as a young kid and loving that, loving teaching and creating. I think we, as adults, get educated out of being creative at work, in the schools and we have a real responsibility to help one another get back to being more creative. I think we're all creative. I don't believe it's an elite genius, I think we all have creativity we just need to find it.

Kevin: That's such an important connection, sharing your creativity or moving it out into the world in its relationship to your internal health.

Robyn: Creativity is part of the solution. I love that message. Janet, a lot of people are experiencing adversity in some shape or another. It seems like this year has been a wowza year. What do you say to someone who's experiencing pain, suffering, adversity or other challenges in life?

Janet: I rolled my sleeves up and I'm doing the same. I'll hopefully lead from example and walk the talk here. Oprah Winfrey and Deepak Chopra have a great 21-day challenge, and you're invited to find ways that you think you are grateful for. One thing I would encourage someone to do if they're going through a tough time and we know the holidays with Thanksgiving and Christmas can be very difficult for many people for a variety of reasons, be it financial or loneliness or depression.

I would invite and encourage them to notice the things that they can be grateful for.

Are they in good health?

Do they value relaxation time?

Can they find something, some way to become passionate towards themselves?

Things like noticing the sunset, getting out and about in their different routines, going to a different restaurant or out to watch a play, finding ways and simple ways they can be truly grateful for and doing that on a daily basis, perhaps writing five different things they're grateful for each day and then doing that. I believe Stephen Covey talked about 21 days to change a habit, so 21 days is a great timeframe to have that.

Robyn: This is a perfect reminder to everyone listening that Janet is our very first speaker of our Pay It Forward month and we're just so grateful to start with your relevant and wonderful message. I just want to remind you that part of the Self-Care Revolution™ journey that many of you have been on is entering the information into your journal. One of the things we ask everyone to consider is writing down 31 things that you can do to Pay It Forward. What ways do you want to wake up in the morning and have this Pay It Forward gratitude ritual? You reminded me of that Janet, as you were speaking, that this call to action is something we've brought into the Self-Care Revolution™ each and every month, so that journal is available in the members area for all of you.

Janet: That's wonderful.

Kevin: Also, because we are in our Pay It Forward month, perhaps you could share some of your stories about paying it forward. In your book you mentioned having a springboard spirit.

Janet: That goes back to the gymnastic metaphor. The springboard spirit is really about the whole mind/body connection and I really believe that towards healing we need to integrate all those in addition to the positive mindset, the gratefulness and being conscious and mindful of the thoughts. The springboard spirit I use as a metaphor in the book and give the visual of, imagine tackling your adversity or challenge and running up to the springboard and taking the leap up and over whatever challenge you're facing.

The gymnast lands on the other side of the springboard and just note that whatever you're going through and experiencing, you have the opportunity to use that once you're beyond it, to share that and springboard and pay that forward as a gift for someone else.

Robyn: I remember when I was reviewing your book you talk about the four pillars. Can you share with the listeners what those are, in terms of the springboard spirit?

Janet: Yes.

    1.   Faith

    2.   Mind

    3.   Body

    4.   Soul

Robyn: How about sharing a little more about soul?

Janet: I'm glad you asked that. I'm not someone who actually grew up around the church and what I had in writing this book was a very spiritual experience, to the point of not really fully understanding what was happening. What I found as I was writing, was I was actually guided and started to pay attention internally in listening to the guidance that I had. So as you read the book you'll see that it's extremely spiritual and it hadn't started out as a spiritual book. I would say it was more of an uplifting positive and inspirational guide, which has turned into a spiritual faith-based book.

With that I would suggest that any of your listeners be open to developing your intuition and be open and obedient to any guidance, whether you get that through prayer or meditation. It's a beautiful experience if you trust it and go with it. I really believe that part of the springboard spirit is integrating the mind, body, soul, and having faith.

Robyn: That's beautiful.

Kevin: You've mentioned many times mindfulness. What is your definition of mindfulness or how do you think people can implement or practice mindfulness in their daily lives?

Janet: If you were to lay back and get into a quiet space, maybe you were laying on your bed and for a lot of people you might experience lots of chatter and you find it difficult to relax and be calm. What I would invite you to do as you close your eyes to relax is to simply notice the different thoughts you're having and instead of holding onto a particular thought. Whether it's irrespective, positive or negative, just imagine yourself as an observer noticing the thoughts you're having but letting them move by on a cloud, just passing you by and literally not being attached to holding on to any particular thought.

Then, in time, choosing which ones you do want to attach and hold onto. I believe many people aren't aware that they can use that part of the brain to really reprogram and have that empowerment, that control, to be able to pay attention and choose which thoughts they want to hang onto and disregard. I think much of that comes from each of our pasts that we've had, maybe the beliefs we've grown up with about who we think we are, according to someone else. It really puts you in a place of empowerment, rather than disempowerment. I think it's important that people realize they have the power to do that and you can set your pattern and the way that you think in a different way.

Robyn: Maybe you can share a little with how exactly you're working with your clients day-to-day and the whole idea of leadership since that's so near and dear to you.

Janet: Absolutely. I actually provide leadership development coaching and personal transformation. I am full on board with servant leadership philosophy and rather actually I would say is a way of being. I am passionate that leaving the corporate world there is a lot of opportunity to improve the health of the environment that we find ourselves working in and it's not until we remove ourselves from those environments that we can actually stand back and see how unhealthy some of the management or leadership that we've been privy to has been and how that's costing companies money, it's increasing insurance costs and people are missing days from work due to stress.

It's affecting people's health and well-being, so I actually coach people that are in transition that are looking to come out of the corporate world. I'm also going into organizations and teaching workshops on servant leadership as a different way of leading, which is all about leading from the heart, leading with compassion and empathy, leading out of humility and really with a sense that we're all connected and that we are coming from a place of serving a grander purpose, a grander mission and not just ourselves.

The leadership development goes back to the heart and I believe that leadership is a heart matter. If we can transform managers, bosses, leaders, people coming out of the corporate world for healing… if we can transition and help them to transform we can cause that ripple effect and we can spread out and help, not just the corporate world, but indeed Pay It Forward and serve each other.

Robyn: I love that.

Kevin: Definitely the transition and transforming and letting that soak in.

Janet: I don't know that it's the most popular style of leadership. I will share with you that I felt as somewhat of a black sheep in the corporate world because I have always led with compassion and empathy, from the heart. I've always cared about people and been connected and helped people from the heart. I think we have a big challenge in the corporate structure to go in and do some amazing work to help transform. There are companies out there that are doing servant leadership and succeeding, like Southwest Airlines, Whole Foods. It's an entirely different way of leading and serving and I'm all on board for that and helping my clients to be better leaders and transform personally.

Kevin: We really are moving away from the direction of competition and into a more cooperative way of running business. I think you are a leader in that and I really like the pyramid on your site, the seven seas of transformation. Those particular words, could you share those with everyone?

Janet: I'm actually not at my computer right now but one of the words is compassion. Having compassion for ourselves and for the people that we work and collaborate with, having that deeper understanding and empathy, recognizing that everybody is different. Everyone has unique talents and gifts and then change, which is huge. Realizing that we're always moving, evolving and recreating and reinventing. Change is inevitable and it's something for having a lasting change there are six or seven key steps to make that happen. We have to be willing and open to change.

As it pertains to the corporate world it's not doing business as usual or as Sir Richard Branson would say, screw business as usual, it's really about leading with compassion, leading from the heart, being open and willing to change and courage. Courage is a big piece of it. It's taking risk. It's being with uncertainty and not knowing what's going to happen next, and finding a way to be with that. Where we are today in this world that is a huge piece, but there's a lot of growth and opportunity that comes with risk taking and having more courage.

Kevin: One of the things you talk about is control and you share a little about what your feeling is about control?

Janet: Control is a perspective. I think people may want to feel like they're in control 100% and I do feel that the reality is that we're not in full control. There are lots of different factors that come into play. With any decision or situation the universe, faith, external situations, etc. we need to focus on what we can control more, things like our attitude, perspective, the controllable rather than those things we can't control, obviously natural things like the weather, natural disasters and things as such. Control is more of an illusion.

Kevin: Speaking of our Pay It Forward month, you've got a wonderful Pay It Forward gift. When folks go to JoinTheSelfCareRevolution.com and login to Janet's speaker page, you'll find the beautiful cover of her book, *A Champions Guide to Thriving Beyond Breast Cancer*. You are offering our listeners today the seven strategies towards healing.

Janet: Yes.

Kevin: Can you speak to what that is?

Janet: I created a healing video. One of the key things in the video as we mentioned earlier was about gratitude and how we can choose to focus on what we can be grateful for each day and if they pick up your journal, didn't you talk about 31 things Robyn?

Robyn: Yes.

Janet: That would be a fabulous way for someone to get started. Instead of focusing on the immediate difficulty or challenge or adversity, try your best to think and notice what you can be grateful for. The climate, the great conversation you had, the person you made smile because of that conversation or the door you held open for someone that needed that. They will get the seven strategies towards healing when they order the book and they also included a free breast cancer resource guide, because I know during a diagnosis it can be stressful and challenging and difficult trying to run around finding all these tools and resources quickly when you need that information at your fingertips yesterday.

Hopefully that will be helpful and give value to either the person diagnosed or their caregiver and family member.

Robyn: That's great and the best website for people to reach you would be what?

Janet: It's JanetIMueller.com.

Robyn: Great. For everyone listening, for anyone who has any questions for us just write to info@jointheselfcarerevolution.com. I have a question for you Janet, something we ask of all our speakers. What does a self-care day look like for you, based on this rich background that you've had and how you're showing up in life as a coach and leader? How do you take care of yourself to keep paying it forward and sharing your message?

Janet: That's a great question and I'll share with you that it has been a challenge in my life as a mom with an eight-year old daughter, so I won't preach to the choir if you will, but I have learned to become better at taking care of me. I think for so many women in particular we go through our day wearing so many different hats and having so many different roles as nurturers, caregivers, lovers that we quite easily can spend so much of our time, as have I in the past, constantly giving and doing and being for others.

So I have come to realize and integrate into my daily routine with a healthy breakfast, a shake and a piece of fruit and I've started to incorporate getting on the treadmill for 35 minutes everyday as best I can. Then usually I'll spend 60 to 90 minutes on personal growth, whether that's meditating or reading to feed my mind, etc. So from the nutrition, exercise, meditation and development, and I'm big on that because if we can start each day and choose to focus on something positive, something simple as John Maxwell, for example, who has those minutes a day with Maxwell motivation videos he does, so for anyone who says I don't have time to read or watch videos, that's a quick fast resource that anyone can use to implement.

Then for those that are driving, they can listen to CDs or something motivational on the way to work. I think encompassing all aspects of self-care is critical.

Robyn: I love that.

Kevin: It's such an inspiration too, because like we said you are a busy person and we can look to this as here's a person that has a busy, multi-faceted life and is still incorporating these simple self-care tactics and techniques.

Robyn: You definitely have a springboard spirit, Janet.

Janet: Thank you. I appreciate that and I hope it serves your listeners and other people. Sometimes a metaphor, whenever faced with a challenge or adversity they can think about that and picture themselves in a meta view if you will, over the obstacle and not to dismiss it but to pay attention to it in order to work their way through it.

Kevin: You have seven daily affirmations that you share in your book. Could you share a few of those with us today?

Janet: Yes. Those you will find in the book on page 29. The springboard spirit seven daily affirmations are...

1. I am keeping my heart desire alive and I will not let my circumstances defeat me.

2. I am courageous and I will keep focused on my heart desires and not let breast cancer stand in my way.

3. I will get up every time if I should fail.

I feel like we have two choices when it comes to life we can either, fall down and forget it or we can check in our attitude and say it didn't turn out the way I wanted, I gave it my best, what's next?

Robyn: I love this approach when you think about cancer and it's not like a war against message. You clearly have a wealth of information between these affirmations and pillars. Just using this metaphor of moving forward and knowing all the possibilities and choices that are out there that this is not necessarily a death sentence. I think it's so important and such a gift that you're giving to so many people.

Janet: I appreciate that Robyn and I thank you for sharing that. I don't really take all the credit at all, because the women in the book clearly demonstrate and share with their story, all different stages of breast cancer and different women from grandmothers to single middle-aged ladies, the whole spectrum. So, while I'd like to take the credit I can't. They all share their stories of courage and hope and collectively, whoever picks up the book whether they have breast cancer or a different kind of cancer and/or if perhaps they're having a challenge or adversity in life, the book will also serve them from a positive mindset and a faith in the springboard spirit.

I feel blessed and grateful to have that out there as a resource for people.

Robyn: I remember you saying early on in our conversation that one out of eight women are being diagnosed with breast cancer. From my understanding it's like one out of four, just being in the medical field. What is correct? I'm so alarmed, like I shared with you before we went live on this call today, one of the big inspirations for me to want to start to be a true revolutionary was the times I had three women in their 30s with breast cancer. That was such a defining moment I'll never forget it. I was like how can this be. I've had a woman in her 20s with breast cancer, so I'm curious about that statistic.

The research that I came across while writing the book, taking a lot from the American Cancer Society, was that one in eight women in their lifetime and I believe that's based on somebody living up to 70 years of age.

Kevin: It's still an appalling figure when we're thinking of eight people that we know.

Janet: Absolutely, and worldwide, I believe it's somewhere close to 1.5 million. I'd love to dive more into the nutrition. We've talked about the mind/body and soul and faith, the whole therapy has me very curious with holistic healing. I'm sure that's right up your alley as well with the nutrition part of cancer.

Robyn: Yes, and the women in your book, what was mostly their nutrition strategy?

Janet: It varied; no one was the same, a very varied approach to nutrition. One girl, Angela, was active. She said she ate fairly healthy for the most part, but then I've spoken to people that have survived cancer that have gone through Gerson therapy's and they've reported healing through the whole organic plant-based juicing diet and the coffee enema's, etc. I think we have a great conversation for another phone call at some point to dive into the whole nutrition part.

Robyn: Yes, we have covered nutrition in a big way in this revolution from brain health to nutrition and exercise to just devoting the very first month. It's such a critical part of the self-care message. We have some of our experts that believe 80% of our health has to do with diet. I'm close to that number. I think it's very important.

Janet: Absolutely. Who was it that said food "be thy medicine?"

Robyn: Hippocrates; "Let food be thy medicine and medicine be thy food."

We're very excited that we'll be interviewing Jeffrey Smith, one of our first speakers in 2014, who will be talking about genetically modified food and talk about a trailblazer. Information is power. Just to know how much of our food supply is genetically modified, so we're excited to have that conversation.

Janet, when you think about where you're going, what are your next steps? You mentioned possibly another book. What's next for Janet Mueller and your big message?

Janet: The big message that I need support with is that I want to get out with the people and create a movement with servant leadership. I see that as a huge healing of hearts and spirits and people of all walks of life, from the corporate world to entrepreneurs. We're all leading in some way, as parents, women, practitioners, we're all leading in some way and we all have those hurts, challenges, wounds and healing from the past to journey through. I truly believe it's a huge calling and message as is yours.

I think together we can probably support each other quite well in getting out there and creating these kinds of movements. There's a lot of healing and hurt and love that's needed in the world. I think servant leadership is the next big piece and hopefully I've demonstrated just a piece of servant leadership with the way that I did the book. I hope that's the message.

Kevin: It definitely resonated with us. Is there a common message that you found in the stories that are shared in your book?

Janet: Great question. One interesting response that I had from many of the women is that having to go through cancer again they would not opt for chemotherapy. That's one common thread that I found. Second, they all had a positive mindset. For the most part their attitudes and outlook on life was mostly positive. Third, is faith. Each of them is a woman of faith.

Kevin: You've said that particular word, Faith, several times in our call. Can you expand upon it and what it means in your life and what you think it really means in the healing process?

Janet: That's a huge question. As a kid I'd always grown up believing in God. I would pray to God. I was not the person that was ever taken to church growing up, but I always prayed and believed. I always knew and felt it in my heart. I think through writing the book there was a healing that happened for me. I think the healing was the missing piece of the Holy Spirit and having been touched by that the way the book unfolded, the women I was led to, the different stages each woman was diagnosed with, I couldn't have planned that as perfect as it turned out.

I think truth be told, my first intent to write a book was going to be all about leadership and that was not the path I was guided down. I think listening and being obedient and trusting what we hear and get and as we connect the dots backwards we can see how it unfolded and perhaps how sometimes it's not our position it's really about listening to what we're supposed to be doing, what we're called to do and following that. I believe that healing happened not only for me without realizing it, but it also happened in videoing the women and having them share their stories on video.

I believe without realizing that they were actually getting healing through not only sharing their stories with me in a journalistic way but they were healing through sharing their message on video as well.

Robyn: That's the Pay It Forward message is energetic transfer without even knowing the power of sharing and how that impacts so many other people's lives, yours and all the readers of the book and those who view the video. That's fantastic.

As we come to the end of our conversation with you. I think we've covered so much. I love the work you're doing. You can feel how tangible your passion for what you're doing is. One final comment based on all this experience and research that you'd like to share with us, regarding getting into the psyche of these women as your wrote the book and practiced leadership and coaching.

Janet: I would say that we need to pay attention all of us, women in particular, to any feelings of bitterness or resentment or any areas in our lives when we may feel we still have some forgiveness to explore and let go of or free ourselves. I think forgiveness is a huge part to healing and I believe when we forgive we are free. I would invite listeners to consider and explore that, to give themselves permission to follow that and find any area or someone whom you feel you may need to forgive. Look at areas where you have existing anger or resentment because I feel that plays a big part towards disease.

I encourage folks to journal and to be grateful for what you can in your life each day. Get Robyn's journal and create those 31 journal entries as well.

Robyn: Love it. Thank you so much for being with us today. For all our listeners we have another wonderful speaker coming soon, Rev. Adara who will follow soon. Thank you for your time and sharing your great story, wisdom and your gift.

Janet: Thank you you're welcome. I appreciate the opportunity. Thanks very much.

[End of Interview]

REV. ADARA WALTON

SpiritIsMyLife.com | Doctor of Naturopathy and PhD in Natural Health, a Bio-Energy Kinesiologist, Certified Quantum-Touch Instructor + Practitioner

HEALING YOUR LIFE WITH BIO-ENERGY KINESIOLOGY

Robyn: Hello everyone, welcome to month 12 of the Self-Care Revolution™ Series where we're literally celebrating 'Celebrate and Pay It Forward'. My name is Robyn Benson. I'm a Doctor of Oriental Medicine and the founder of Santa Fe Soul Health and Healing Center. When it comes to this Pay It Forward message, what I love to do is share my 21 years of experience as a Doctor of Oriental Medicine with each and every client I see, patient, a friend, family member, to help people achieve optimal health. I am joined today with...

Kevin: Kevin Snow. I am an Intuitive Counselor at Santa Fe Soul. My Pay It Forward message is to help people create clarity in their lives and I am very grateful to have one of my fellow practitioners and amazing gifts to Santa Fe Soul, Reverend Adara, with us today.

Robyn: Reverend Adara certainly is that. What a treasure we get to share you and I'd love for you to share a story of how we met once upon a time. Just for all of you listening live with us right now, I am here at Santa Fe Soul, Adara is at her brand new home, Kevin is in Arizona and I was just sitting in the kitchen looking over our 12 months of this series and all the speakers who had different themes starting out with Thoughts and Food as Medicine, month three where we celebrated Transmuting and Releasing Trauma, we just finished Gratitude Month and here we are at Pay It Forward and I'm like wow!

This message has been so powerful and we are so grateful to all of you listening live with us now and all of our members. We literally have people from many different countries and we just say thank you for many of you being here and choosing self-care as a way of life and following this series and knowing that this is so exciting because now it's Pay It Forward time. How does that sound to everybody?

Kevin: Great.

Robyn: Sounds great, ha? Well, Miss Adara, Reverend Adara Walton, is an ordained Reverend, Doctor of Naturopathy and Ph.D. in Natural Health, a Bio-Energy Kinesiologist, Certified Quantum-Touch Instructor and Practitioner, Reiki/Amanohuna master teacher/practitioner, Shaman and Certified Attractor Field Technique Practitioner. For 25 years she used Aromatherapy, Homeopathy, color and vibrational remedies. She is the author of *Truth: Muscle Testing for the Masses* with Shamanic journey odyssey into light.

Welcome Adara.

Adara: Hello there. Hi to everyone in the audience, everyone listening and especially to Kevin and to Robyn.

Robyn: I have to say it's always so uplifting just hearing your voice and being live with you always puts a smile on my face. It's just been great to have you as a wonderful addition to our Santa Fe Soul community. For any of you that are here with us for the very first time, as we mentioned, the Self-Care Revolution™ has been going on 12 months as a series and the home of the Self-Care Revolution™ is Santa Fe Soul Health and Healing Center where we have over 25 practitioners and offer over 50 different services. We are not only practitioners, but also self-care coaches here to serve you – small or large, whatever issues you may have now that we are a phone call away.

So Adara, you've got quite an interesting topic today and that is, basically, sharing your history of working as a Bio-Energy Kinesiologist. For people who are joining us for the first time or may not know what that is, could you just give us a history of this session title Healing Your Life With Bio-Energy Kinesiology, how you got into it and your pathway to becoming a Practitioner, Healer, Naturopathic Doctor, Reverend and all the above?

Adara: Okay. That was a mouthful, but a journey that has been similar I think to a lot of people's in terms of having your own health challenges and how do you find something like Bio-Energy Kinesiology and what that really is. I came to it years ago because, basically, I got tired of getting what I call 'disempowered' by your conventional doctors. Even as a young woman, I got tired of going in and getting poked and probed. They had gone to school to tell me what was wrong with me and how I was out of balance and it just felt really disempowering in a couple cases, which I won't share with the audience. I was literally insulted in this doctor's office and I'm laughing because I can look back over what used to be painful times and laugh about it at this point in my life now, but it brought me into what I call this act of service and I'll spend a sentence or two on that.

Basically, Bio-Energy Kinesiology is a field. Some people may be familiar with it. It used to be called Specialized Kinesiology. A lot of people have heard of basic Kinesiology, which is the movement and study of muscles. You have people that do rehabilitative services with that, but Energy Kinesiology is exactly that. It's the study of the movement of energy in the body. I know a lot of your other speakers have talked about how we are energetic beings. We're magnetic, we're electric and, therefore, we are electromagnetic as human beings, but we do go in and out of balance based on our thoughts, based on the cosmology of who we are spiritually. We go in and out of balance based on the foods we eat, what we drink. There's so much variation between what you eat, what you absorb, what you think. All of those are actually correct answers.

I don't disagree or separate myself from clients when I'm doing this work, but basically, the Bio-Energy field is exactly that. It's a field. It's the study of energy and the movement within the body and it is designed to take stress off the body at whatever level it is. So we can look at categories, which we often do. We look at the person holistically. This is a holistic field, so we do look at the person spiritually. I look at the person on a physical level. I also look at them emotionally. We look at the psychological or what are called the mental energy balance level. We also look at the person, if we have to look at past life, what I call karmically. So you get a whole total picture and that is why I had to study different modalities to help me with the service that I give to people doing the study of Bio-Energy Kinesiology.

I would like to state that almost any issue--and I'm not trying to be what I call the Jack of all trades here, but almost any issue that causes stress in the body can be addressed by having what we call a balance/diffusion session. So if you have it, if there's something and you're off in let's say your meditations, your prayers, your rituals, whatever that is, then that's the spiritual category that can be addressed. A lot of us have issues with relationships, whether it's your significant other, whether it's marital or whatever, that may call for relationship balance. Again, we're looking at stress on the system, not what's wrong with the person. We're looking at an energetic imbalance and where it is. So is it emotional? Is it spiritual? Is it simply physical?

In the service that I do and I do like to call it service instead of work because I use the art of what's called muscle testing biofeedback to access the responses needed to take the stress off the body wherever it is. So that's kind of in a nutshell what a balance session is. Now, how long it is depends on the work that's being done. My normal session is anywhere between 45 to 60 minutes to actually balance and issue and it doesn't matter how long your body energetically has held it. It could have held it from past lives. It could actually hold an issue for 25, 30-40 years and often people just don't believe. Can you really balance a session, can you take stress off in one session and my answer is an emphatic yes, you can.

I've been doing it for over 20-some years and very rarely do I see a person for the same stressor twice. The reason for that being, if the person comes back, they usually have not done what I call the home reinforcement. With all of the balance session I do there is a component at the very end. I don't like the word homework. Again, most of us didn't like homework in school, so you either did it or you struggled with it. But that word 'work' actually will weaken the body when you do a muscle test on it, so we don't use the word work. We say home reinforcement and that's kind of a nice middle-of-the-road word that the body really does like.

Actually, any issue can be addressed in these sessions. It doesn't matter if it's weight reduction. I actually have a specific balance for weight. Some people want to weigh a certain amount. Well, I will look at what is it you would like to weight and then we ask the body what it would like to weigh and then we support that with a nutritional balance. So that does mean looking at the foods you eat, it means looking at perhaps adding supplements or changing the supplements and I do deal with the emotional.

I have found that almost every disorder or disease has an emotional component to it, which is why a lot of our modalities…I won't say that they don't work, but if people don't follow through and if they don't address the holistically as a whole (w-h-o-l-e) then what happens is you're only addressing one part of what I call that three-legged, four-legged stool. If something is showing up on a physical level as a disease, as a disorder, you need to find the root of the issue and that is the heart of my work or service.

The reason I like to call it service and I'm sure a lot of the speakers you've had on, we don't look at this perhaps as work. At least speaking for myself, I don't. I feel that I am working with a person not on a person and I also feel that what I'm doing, even though I had to learn this professionally and study under many teachers and even travel the world learning my techniques. It is a service. A service is something you render to another human being and you do it because you love it.

People have asked me, would I do this if I didn't get paid and the answer is yes. I think you've seen while I've been at Santa Fe Soul I'm always trying to assist here and I'm not asking for money. Money is just one component and, for instance, if I need it I can do what's called a financial re-patterning. I do have a balance with people that are holding. Again, it's an energetic based on perhaps what your parents felt, others around you, your friends, your colleagues, what they thought about money.

We incorporate a lot of collective things in our subconscious and so my work actually does go to the subconscious level to take stress off there, to take things off, because who wants to have an issue in their life. Most of us don't, but if we don't have something to test our metal supposedly with and to walk the walk, you don't have the strength with which to address other things.

So there is a reason we have the challenges, but when they get so what I call surmountable that they start to cause undue stress and put us in overwhelm that's when we attract the disease or the disorder that tends to match emotionally what is going on, on the subconscious level. So again, anything can almost be addressed and that includes: opiates and even addictions. You can do this work through getting a balance session or a diffusion using Bio-Energy Kinesiology. I'll stop with that.

Kevin: I don't know about you, Robyn, but this is why we call her Reverend Adara. I could listen to her as an orator just all day long.

Robyn: Both of us have been practitioners for quite some time, too, I mean the wealth of experience, Adara, you bring to the table to be able to bring all your amazing jewels together from bringing in Aroma Therapy to the Kinesiology to all your other toys, I call them, because I have some, too. For example, I have a pharmacy of at least 28 different companies and I love it when she goes in with this tester. She can actually determine the vitality that remains in that particular supplement or that's innate in it. Some of these products are not even expired, they just don't have vitality.

Going back to all that you've shared so far, the body is pretty complicated. You were talking about all these different systems, the mental, the physical, the chemical, the emotional, you're integrating all that to really get to the root problem that's causing the physiological effects that might be showing up in the body, the depression, the whatever. I think it's great. I think we all need some balancing in today's world. What do you think, Kevin?

Kevin: We definitely do and I think that Reverend Adara is bringing it back to our topic this month of paying it forward by identifying the work that she does as an act of service. I do think we all have a service that we can provide to the world and use that to Pay It Forward into the world.

Adara: Yes. Again, we all have these fields of work we do. We all have whatever drew us to our particular field, but I really think for what I call Pay It Forward or even forward thinking. To even change our own consciousness, we have to look at what we bring to our work. We bring our heart to these fields. We bring our hearts to the service we are rendering. When you really look at it, again, as service, regardless of what ailment you're trying to take off with whatever modalities we are all trained to use, if we don't approach any of this, if I don't approach even my diffusion sessions, my Bio-Energy Kinesiology, if I don't approach it with love, with a real genuine devotion in my heart to really help, I'm not going to help someone to the degree that I would want for help.

I can feel something when clients leave after a session. When they're satisfied, when their heart is full, I can feel those dynamics in my session. Even people who don't know what this is, the trust level gets build up and I think that's between any practitioner, any facilitator. As I've said, I work with people, I don't work on them. The body will unfold its truth, and that's why I wrote my book *Everybody's Truth: Muscle Testing for the Masses*, because the truth is within all of us. All I do with the work that I'm doing, this field of practice, is unlocking the truth and taking the stress off so you can absolutely unfold and be the optimal human being you can be.

Some of us are graced to walk a path which looks like suffering, what looks like pain, but at the root of it you cannot identify with that on the physical level or even emotional. That's why I talk about these five levels that my work delves into. This field has to take the stress off that so as you unpeel the onion, unpeel all those stresses, unpeel all the layers, you reach the pearl, the heart, the gem of that person. As a Reverend, I do believe that we're still created in that image of spirit. So whatever it is we are graced to have, whether you are beset with whatever it is called, it is a learning process. It is something that we can take the stress off of and once we learn from it, sometimes, healing is our calling. It is all self-healing. That's on my website, all healing is self-healing.

Sometimes we cannot heal on this side of the veil, as I call it. The healing has to be done on another side on another level and that's when I get into past life when I do have to look at is this karmic disorder that is visiting the person and, again, taking the stress off. What do we need to learn from this, can it be resolved in this lifetime on this side of the veil or is this a purpose that this person has to carry forward and do on another side. So we do look at that. That's where my Sharman training comes in, as Kevin well knows. He has to visit this work, also. We look into the soul of the person and that is not exactly the same as the spirit, but there can be stress even on those levels and so we take that off because the spirit of a person really is in its Divine perfection.

I'm not going to say that I don't have my druthers or expectations when I'm doing a session with someone because I can feel, I can see, the other gifts that I've asked of the Holy Spirit, God, whatever word you use for God. I don't let that separate my clients from the session and what we're doing, but all my work is done with permission from what I call the highest level. My training and my techniques yes, as I've said, I've had to go around the world. I've had to study with several people. I've had to get the hard core what I call academic degrees. But all of that aside, what I'm looking at is helping another child of God to unfold their beauty, to unfold their Divine purpose for why they are walking on this planet at this time.

I don't feel that we have to walk in undue stress and pain for an inordinate amount of time and even victimize ourselves and that's what some of us do. We have so many evaluations, so many criticisms that are put upon us and we adopt those, but we're not those things. We were talking about that at the staff meeting. We're not those collective thoughts. We're not everything. We may be a composite, but it's what you select to own. If there's stress trying to own something that isn't yours, we need to take the stress off. We need to take any negativity out, unless you can learn I don't have to be negative about something.

I learned long ago to walk through negativity, not run from it. I used to try to do that when I was younger, go around it. I have to now on a mental level examine why did I engage that, did I help create it, but I don't have to own it so that I can really release that and take all the stress off so that I can smile and it takes less and less, of course, to smile, so that I can be my perfect self, so that I can be of service and have a genuine devotion to my family, my friends, those that I love and in return you get that love back.

So, yes, as I tell people, I love what I do and, yes, I would do it without being paid. That's just the real truth because, for me, one of the highest services you can do is to be of service. You have to settle that within yourself, but people see that within someone like Kevin as a practitioner and Robyn, that kind of devotedness that you all have. I love when I came there the name Santa Fe Soul, because there's a soul not just in the name, there's something alive in it. That same aliveness that chi, that vitality, is what I have to reawaken with my clients by just taking any of this stress off.

We look at our children, there's stress with their nutrition. There's this bullying that goes on in school. How do you stop that? Sometimes you have to look at the child who is doing it. What is their emotional need? What created the need to have to do that again? My work will go to the root of any issue and, with the techniques, makes an attempt to take the stress off wherever it is. Once you do that, the body does know how to heal itself and it likes to try to go back to a state of homeostasis and balance.

Kevin: Yes!

Robyn: Yes!

Kevin: I love this.

Robyn: You know what? We really are being generous with Adara. We're letting her talk because, again, there's so much information in every sentence.

Kevin: You touched on several different modalities that you do. Obviously, I'm very interested in the Shamanic path and working with the soul, but that is an aspect of all of the work that you do. I know that you have a class coming up, is it this weekend?

Adara: Thank you Kevin. Yes, most of what I've talked about is on the bio-energetic level, but it was mentioned that I also do something called Quantum Touch, which is another healing modality. In fact, my dissertation was actually dealing with clients with chronic musculoskeletal pain and relief using what is called Quantum Touch Healing. That's a system that was developed by Bob Rasmussen and then when he made transition passed on to one of his students Richard Gordon.

I actually am a Certified Instructor. I will be teaching that class in 2014. There are two levels, a beginning and an advanced level. That is dealing with hands-on as well as what we call remote and long-distance healing. It actually relieves pain from the body. You can actually see the bones moving in the body with touch or without touch.

Again, it's a very satisfying field to come in and in seconds adjust someone's hip and then watch the head move or the pain just simply dissolve and release from the body.

The class I'm teaching this Sunday at Santa Fe Soul is in the sunroom from 1:00 to 4:00. It is a Reiki class. I do have seven different Reiki Masterships. I do teach four different styles of Reiki. Reiki, again, is a form of noninvasive, but it's hand-on healing. Again, if there's a laceration, a burn or an area that can't be touched, with Reiki you can also send what we call remote, long distance. Some people call it Tele Reiki.

The Reiki class I'm teaching this Sunday is one that has not been seen very much, even in this area or even in the State of Maryland. Most people think of Reiki when they think of western Reiki or Usui Reiki. They think of Karuna. I am also a Karuna Master. Kathleen Nagy, another wonderful staff person, we call her the sound lady, she would love that form, because it uses the voice and toning with which to do healing, but you also use the hands. This particular Reiki class, however, is the simplest, what I call the easiest to teach. It is the most gentle. You do not need equipment and that's why I love this one.

This form of Reiki can be taught to anyone that has never had any Reiki, doesn't know what it is. For instance, you do not need a table, you don't need a bolster, and all you need are your hands and chairs. We do use a pendulum in the class, but even to learn that is an easy class. I have a class that I teach on that and it's only an hour and a half. The way I use the pendulum, the way I learned it from Hanna Kroger, is a little bit different than what most people use, but this particular one is called Kundalini Reiki. For people who are interested, I do want them to know, no, I do not open up your Kundalini. I do not open that pathway.

Robyn: Bummer.

Adara: We don't do that. It just happens to be called Kundalini Reiki because this form of Reiki does the cleansing of the Kundalini as you learn it, but it does it in increments. There are long-distance attunements that are sent for this class and it culminates in learning the actual physical technique and that's what we will do this Sunday. It's the shortest Reiki class that I teach compared to my other classes that are about 10 to 11 hours long and require at least a couple of days. This is simply a three-hour class.

With your heart and with your desire to be of service, if you have one chair in your apartment or house or whatever, you can actually learn Reiki and administer Kundalini Reiki. Again, it's the simplest, easiest form to use and is still what I call the laying on of hands. It is very gentle and the client simply sits in the chair to receive it. So that's the first of my classes that I'm going to offer at Santa Fe Soul and I am just so happy that I'm a part of this community.

Kevin: That again, goes right along with our Pay It Forward message. There are people that have these healing gifts, we all do, and the way you're boiling this down for us I think is so important. This is something that can be taught. There is a piece of this that can be taught. There is a piece of this that is your heart that you share with others. Truly, the Pay It Forward message is when we have some of these modalities in our toolkit, even if we don't believe we're a healer, we can help people in our lives in very profound ways.

Adara: Yes, people don't look at really the gift. God, the Holy Spirit, is allowing all of these gifts we all have to come out. This is the cosmology, this community, of each one teach one. Each one has to help one. For you to think you're just self-reliant and independent, I really just laugh at that. You may be in a space by yourself or alone, but that's not the cosmology of where we're headed right now. This is community and living in communities. I live here in my house, but my community is now Santa Fe Soul. My community is new people that I'm meeting. My community is the clients and the children of the Most High that I'm serving and in doing so I am serving myself. So this is a nice and easy, especially the class Sunday what I call a Pay It Forward.

I remark about a book I read, that the gifts that we really have are within. You will look at something and you think it has to be special. It has to be recognized by some authority outside of what I call your God Presence and it doesn't. The mere fact that you were self-created, you have a gift or gifts within. Again, that's what my work likes to do with the Kinesiology, take the stress off so you can see what it is. Because all of us, including me, there is something that I know I can't do or I won't do, but I will pay someone or barter with someone to do.

I remember *Do What You Love,* it's a book and it was one of the ones that inspired me that feel into my possession. Do what you love and the money will follow. There are a lot of people with careers or doing things that they got a degree for, but it doesn't really make them happy. I walked away from that myself and I've seen a lot of people do that, why? Your heart isn't in it. Love is something that has to touch. Again, it's about gifting, it's about service and so what you draw to yourself or what you still in your own strength encourage will say I am going to pursue that because that's what my devotedness is, that's what my real service is.

Okay, so I got the degree. I did this and did that. Is that going to bring you not even happiness, is it going to bring you joy. So look at what it is you're doing in your life. Look at your career if it's something that you want to pursue. I've done this so many years with what is called a career balance. I actually have a session and it's called A Career Balance and what it does is it addresses out and out changing the career path. If you don't think I had balance with myself, I did, because that is one of the things that got me on this path.

This is so funny, but I had a lack of confidence in doing this work. About 20-some years ago, one of my teachers said you are just relentless and I was just very dogged. I didn't know what it was inside me, but it was this passion. It was this drive to be of servicing doing something different. That just fuels me, but I had a lack of confidence when I was learning meridians, when I was learning the chakras, the colors, the tones and the sounds. If you think I wasn't putting everything in a hodgepodge and messing it up, but something and I found out what that is. Now, it wasn't a something. It was really what I had come to call the God Presence within was fueling me to be of service, to make me be passionate about the gifts and discover what is it I wanted to give to people, what is it I wanted to service with humanity with dignity, with respect and with real high techniques.

So that's what drove me into this field and to travel the world to study with other people, other healers, even to learn, Kevin mentioned, Shamanism. There's an aspect of that where I really get into the spiritual level of a person, the soul level of a person. When you find that there's such stress, such trauma, Dr. Robyn talked a few minutes ago about dealing with the shock and trauma and we had speakers addressing that. Well, when you have it to the point that even a part of that person flees, it goes into a very, very deep retreat at the subconscious level and the person consciously doesn't even know what they're exhibiting or their disorder or their discomfort or their melancholy. They don't know that it's stemming from this part. The soul is just crying out for help, but you've got to go find what level it's on. Where is the loss and how do bring that back into the person, how do you bring it back incrementally.

I remember the first time I actually did one of these soul what I call soul retrievals. The person had lost a great amount of their childhood and we when finished the session, these sessions for me normally take 90 minutes their not what I call bio energy kinesiology, it's Shamanic work. It's very high spiritual work and it's not what I call for the faint of heart you really have to have yourself pretty well organized and strong within, because some of the things, as Kevin knows, we come up against and I say other energies we come up against in these kinds of sessions.

Again, nothing can repay the satisfaction that you feel when you see part of that intelligence part of that person's soul come back into them. I remember one in particular, a woman for about a week afterwards, because she had no recollection between about three or four per years her very young childhood was gone. She had also been put out as a teenager and it's the only soul retrieval where I literally went in looking for one part and two parts came back. A child at three years old came back and this teenager at fourteen and the teenager at fourteen helps me go find the child at three. It was one of the most miraculous soul retrievals that I did.

For about a week after the woman all she wanted to do was eat ice cream, eat candy and do all these, children can we go to the zoo and I'm like what is she asking us to do. It was the body's response to the missing childhood, to the missing pleasures; to the things that children do that they love. So I said go out and do it do whatever I don't care your fifty something years old go to the zoo. I know what the sugar and all that does, but we're talking about a temporary, the body was calling for, give me the sweetness that was missing from my life as a child. So I said just go do it what's a week going to do as opposed to all the other things? Nothing.

The impact to her soul, to her heart and to putting her back together as a whole human being, which is the work that I do whether its Reiki or quantum touch, all of that seeks to put you back together in that wholeness. For me, you can hear it in my voice, I get very passionate about it even when I'm talking about what I do in the sessions with people but to see the wholeness, the satisfaction, to see the smiles, to see the light and as we say we are created in the image of spirit. God is spirit and there's light. You are created in image of light and that is one of the very basic techniques that I teach almost every client without exception.

I don't care if their children I've taught from two years old, teenagers or adults. You carry a light within you as part of that vitality and the chi force and most of us have not be trained most practitioners, I don't care what modality it is, we have not been trained to access that light which is such a vial part of our spirit and our soul. So, I teach people how to raise their light whether I do an energy kinesiology technique or Reiki. When you even take the word apart key the oriental you can call it Rei-chi it doesn't matter, chi vitality, key life force, energetic life force, it has to be feed by the light.

We look at the processes of photosynthesis and look at the light I mean I could go on about Jacob Leiberman and his book and the studies that have been done with light on plants and food. What do you think is happening to our children when they're in school and can't learn they have these learning issues? What do we do we label them. If we would simply change the lighting in the home by the bulb and use what we call full spectrum light, and I try to put them in the house that I'm in now because they enhance your vitality.

I could continue forever with my passion, so I'm going to stop just now to see if there's something else you want to talk about. It's a gift and devotedness that I have. I don't want to neglect, even before finishing the interview, I do want to say how I found this path was I prayed, that was the very first thing that I did over 25 years ago. At that point I thought I had to get on my knees, whereas I don't have to now, but at that time I got on my knees and I have space always devoted to creative, Source, God, whatever name you call it. I have space, so at that time I simply got on my knees and said how can I be a real service to humanity? How can I be of service to my people? What is it you want me to do God? I asked from the depths of my heart, because at that time I had two degrees and was working what I call a good government job and I was most dissatisfied with my life.

I said I am not making a difference I don't care if I have a house and a car. I'm not making a difference in my life. I'm not making a difference in someone else's life? How am I going to feel whole? So I prayed from the very center, the depth of my heart and I waited for an answer, which happened to come during that particular meditation. I felt blessed, because sometimes I have to wait myself, longer for answers. Sometimes I have to wait for the responses with my clients. The one thing I get from my heart satisfaction is in doing these sessions, regardless of which work it is you work with me, it doesn't matter. When we're doing them we're in this together and I'm going to do my utmost to get you back to being the divine person that you are really here for, so you can get about your purpose, discover your gifts and then you can Pay It Forward to someone else.

That is what this is about, for me.

Robyn: We all need to breathe. I think when you think about the keys to the kingdom so to speak, of health and wellness, it's so broad but if you would comment on two or three things that are critical for people to not only achieve optimal health but radiant and sustainable health.

Adara: Yes. First of all I think, and I will use those words because this part does come from my head, but part is really about ingesting. We do so much with nutrition, but I want to go one step beyond that because the power of the mind and heart when they're linked together, and I think of my work with HeartMath and dressing stress with children who are labeled ADD and ADHD and how you calm them down bringing peace to the heart and mind.

The one message I want to tell people is I really want desire that people watch their thoughts and mend the mind, but before we mend the mind I'd rather just mind the mind. Mind your brain. What are the thoughts? There's a spiritual book that I'm sure people are familiar with, but how many people have really read it, *As a Man Thinketh; As a Woman Thinketh,* so is he/she. Thoughts are things and oftentimes the power of what you are thinking can create and manifest. People don't look at the words I am and then whatever follows it, the blank that follows it. I'm sick and tired of… I'm such and such… you will, because those words carry a spiritual energy with them and whatever follows those words, I am… at some point it will manifest in your life on a physical level.

The one gem I would like, even before we talk about water and nutrition and what you're feeding your body, most of which is water and drinking water, especially the right kind of water for you, which is secondary. It's those thoughts that we have because those thoughts are things and biblically, for those who study the Bible, the Koran or any of those books. The power of life and death is in the tongue. We talk about speaking a word over someone, but what are you speaking in your own life? What are you speaking to yourself to yourself at a high level?

What you speak around yourself and inside your mind, not necessarily being verbal, what you're thinking I would like people to monitor their thoughts and keep them health and positive. Even if it is a negative thought cancel it. I tell people we're in this age of technology, what happens when you make a mistake on the computer when typing something in? You just backspace and delete it, so if you look at your brain as being a computer then you can do the same thing with it. If a negative thought enters monitor it and take it out, delete it, just say cancel. Omit. Whatever it might be just replace it with a healthy high positive thought and watch how you can transform your body physically and emotionally on different levels.

Robyn: That's great. It's interesting you mention the book *Do What You Love the Money Will Follow*, because when I was only 23 and had just moved to Santa Fe being so confused after college, wondering what I wanted to do with my life, that was the first book I bought in downtown Santa Fe.

Adara: Isn't that interesting.

Robyn: I thought that helped me develop that healthy mindset that I can do what I love to do and have a healthy income doing that. It was pivotal. People get really ticked off by that book too.

Adara: Yes.

Robyn: It might be a schoolteacher or something else and they're like I'm doing what I love to do but I'm not making the money I want. So it's interesting you brought that book up. I didn't know that we shared that interest.

Adara: Yes. The second one I'd like, and it's still about words. I just addressed that at the staff meeting last night, cosmology and we use so many words and talk from such a psychological mental intellectual level, but we have to distill this into feeling, so the second book that was pivotal to me that I know God put in my hands was *Feel the Fear and Do It Anyway*. I'm telling you, I was the worst one when I was first studying these classes and having to get the degrees and I know we all have memories of academic pain, but what kept me was when that book and they fell right behind each other.

I couldn't believe it, they were like my little bibles with my third Bible, because I thought okay if I'm serving I have to push on and move what is moving me, so at least I have that identified but I was botching it up as I say on the physical level, because I was going to work, going to school and then I was taking these classes because something was pushing me to go another way.

What is this passion? My heart is pushing me another way and I have no choice, which was my choice. I don't want to say no choice, because no choice is also a choice, when you choose not to do something. I chose to move forward but I did have at that time a fear. You're either in the camp of fear or you really are in the camp of love, so I said how am I going to do this? *Feel The Fear and Do It Anyway.* So yes, I had a fear that I wasn't going to learn everything I wanted. I was going to screw up running someone's meridian the incorrect way. I was not going to learn a hydration technique that takes me 20 minutes to do and I finally got it down to 10.

I had another balance that used to take me an hour and I finally got that down to 30 minutes, but I was relentless and dogged in my determination, because what over rolled my fear was that I want to serve. I love humanity and I have got to do this for me, for my own salvation, for my own love for myself. So I felt the fear, false expectation appearing real, that's what it means. So yes, I was feeling it in my body and was making it real. I wasn't monitoring my thoughts and when I decided to put myself in that position the higher self, the presencing of God within me moved me to a different level and said feel it, embrace it and love it and love it out of your body.

That is when I embraced the excellence in this work, in this fullness and everything became simple and easy, which his why I love what I do.

Kevin: One of the questions we ask all our speakers Adara is what does a self-care day look like in your life? How do you start your day, integrate or incorporate all these things you've shared with us today?

Adara: One of the very first things I do is what I call accessing and practicing the presence. I cannot do anything without accessing what I call the God presence within me, so one of the very first things I do is actually meditate. I do distinguish and also pray. I distinguish meditation and prayer separate for me. I know this isn't a venue to discuss it, but I want to say for me they are different.

The first things I actually do is arise and meditate first. I give thanks for another day. I give thanks for another breath. I give thanks for things like Santa Fe Soul coming to me, the gifts the people have, their friendship and everything. I have to do that and I did a lot of that around Thanksgiving. Even the preceding days and days after of giving thanks and being grateful, that's another way to Pay It Forward. Being grateful for the stumbling blocks in your life or whatever it is. That's one of the first things I do.

Then, I attempt to take care of what I call my physical needs. There is a five-minute routine. Donna Eden, who is another colleague of mine, has a wonderful book out on bio energy kinesiology and she has a five-minute routine, where you can do a crown stretch, which activates the crown chakra in your brain. I do what I call tapping, one of the other of my fields is AFT, which is attract or feel technique. Many people are familiar with EFT, which I also do, but that's a little tapping to wake up the brain.

There are two basic meridians and I always run my central and governing. I teach parents to do that for children because when they have nightmares if you take care of those two meridians and instill the light, which is a short technique, you can set a child on their daily path and ready for school being in a much better frame of mind than the way we send them off by okay, you just want to do the nutrition. That's not enough. We are spiritual and energetic beings and it's time that all of us, parents and practitioners, that we learn to address the other invisible subtle levels in our lives, for ourselves and in our children.

I would do the meditation first. If I'm asked and moved to do some prayer I am always praying. I get requests via email from friends and colleagues to do prayer. There's something in the way that I pray and I have a prayer team, so I turn it over not as just me but as a collective. I either meditate and I'm doing prayers and I will separate those as need be. Then I address my physical by doing the five-minute routine to wake my brain up so I'm not lethargic. I always feed myself light. I have to surround myself in that light and I do that also before I go to bed as well as upon waking after the meditation.

After I do the energetic routine and the meditations that's when I seek what I call physical sustenance. I drink structured water in the morning and there's a small meal that I do to keep my body alkalized. I don't eat food or breakfast in the morning. I will eat almonds that have soaked overnight to alkalize my body. I drink alkaline water as well as another structured water and I don't allow myself to eat until I know that has taken effect and then I eat a very small meal. I love to eat but that's not what sustains me. If I don't have a client to work with or a session then I will do some reading.

Right now because I'm finishing my last Doctorate in Theocentric Psychology, a divinity degree for which I'm doing a lot of reading and I have about 12 books that I have to go through. I feed myself what I call the Word so I can get through this next degree. I'm not really a lunch person so after reading I might do an early morning breakfast and then eat a larger meal. I'm trying to train my body to eat before a certain time because I know in women if we eat after a certain time our bodies are different in terms of other needs so we have to eat differently. I notice my sleep pattern is affected by the time that I eat.

Therefore, I try to eat organically and healthily. If I do eat what I call meats or poultry it's still going to be natural, organic. My day has at least three, and this is 7 days a week, maybe four times for meditation/prayer during what I call the Easter season, for advent I do a little bit more and that's because there are special energies that are upon the earth on Mother Gaia at that time, so I like to feed into that so I may do some chanting and some other collective things.

That's my routine day. When I'm working with clients I love that so when I'm finished with clients and my day then I do a little process of taking the energy off myself, usually after I leave Santa Fe Soul or when I get home. Again, that's another energy process so that you don't retail anything that you may have engaged in so you don't take home a person's grief, sadness, anger or whatever it is. Because you are working in someone's field and sometimes they can trigger similar issues that you had, so I have a process of taking the energy off myself. At least once a month I do take what is called "a spiritual bath", which is to keep the spiritual level of me in hand so I'm still receptive.

Oftentimes I do get information clairvoyantly or auditorily of how to help a client and work with them. If I'm nurturing myself, not just physically but also spiritually, that keeps me open to the highest level in intelligence within me, to help someone else. That's what my day looks like.

Kevin: Wow! That's awesome. We all appreciate that. We have wrapped up another hour.

Robyn: I am amazed. I always love hearing all of these ways in which you are a messenger and amazing healer. You walk your talk and that's felt in your presence always. We're grateful to have you here sharing with our self-care revolutionaries and all those that have chosen this pathway to live a fun, fulfilled and engaged life and to Pay It Forward.

Kevin: Absolutely.

Adara: I thank both of you from my heart for allowing me to come speak to you and your audience, because you have such other people that have such great gifts and so much to share. I'm deeply humbled that I could even have a few words to say today.

Robyn: Fantastic! For everyone listening, be sure to join us for our next special guest Marcella Vonn Harting, who will be sharing the deep healing affects of essential oils. She has traveled around the world many times with founder Gary Young and she has quite an amazing story to share. The rest of the month includes amazing speakers. Thank you Adara for being with us. Thank all of you for listening.

Kevin: Absolutely. Thank you Rev. Adara for sharing your acts of service and paying it forward to our Self-Care community.

Robyn: Everyone take care and have a fabulous day. We look forward to you joining us again at the Self-Care Revolution™.

[End of Interview]

MARCELLA VONN HARTING

MVonn.com | PhDc, Internationally Recognized Author, Speaker, Facilitator, And Entrepreneur, Royal Crown Diamond In Young Living Essential Oils

SELF-CARE AND SUCCESS WITH ESSENTIAL OILS

[These statements have not been evaluated by the Food and Drug Administration. The information on this audiocast is not intended to diagnose, treat, cure, or prevent any disease.]

Robyn: Hello everyone and welcome to month twelve of the Self-Care Revolution™. We have this exciting theme, Pay It Forward, and we're having a blast so far. My name is Robyn Benson. I'm a Doctor of Oriental Medicine and the Founder of Santa Fe Soul Health and Healing Center and I have been loving this co-creation process of the Self-Care Revolution™. I jus want to say a big gratitude to all of you who have been with us since the very beginning.

What a year it has been. Talk about paying it forward, we have literally over 100 speakers who have been with us, our live streams with the Self-Care coaches and this is the greatest opportunity of all, the end of this year to get this message out to literally a billion people, which is our mission and knowing that it will save millions of lives. It will help people not only prevent but also reverse disease and live an engaged, fun and fulfilled life everyday. I'm joined by…

Kevin: Kevin Snow, an Intuitive Counselor at Santa Fe Soul and a Shamanic practitioner. We are going to have a blast this month. Coming out of gratitude and moving into this Pay It Forward is going to be incredible. We're grateful to have Marcella Vonn live on the call today. Welcome Vonn.

Vonn: Thank you very much.

Robyn: It's so great to have you here. I'm going to say that I'm very fortunate to know Vonn as a dear friend and I so admire the work she's doing in the world and has been doing for over 20 years. I was also fortunate to meet Gary Young last December, a year ago. Hopefully, you've all had the opportunity to watch the short video. I actually got him live, and just to hear him speak about his affiliation with the self-care movement for over 30 years as he says, and he's traveled the world many times over to offer this great product to all of us, oils. Talk about self-care.

I can't think of a better person to interview than my dear friend Vonn Harting, just to hear her wealth experience, not only with oils but also in the self-care movement and all that she offers. Let me share a little bit about Vonn.

Marcella Vonn Harting, PhD is an internationally recognized author, speaker, facilitator, and entrepreneur. Involved in the industry since the 1980's, Marcella Vonn has built two highly successful distributorships with more than 250,000 representatives worldwide. In her Leadership Play Shops she demonstrates how creating a residual abundant income centered in health and wealth can empower balance and purpose in one's life.

Marcella Vonn has lectured throughout the United States, Canada, Europe, Australia, Japan, Mexico, and Malaysia. She combines nutrition, conscious communications, face and body language into her dynamic presentations to assist people in creating the life of their hearts desires and dreams. With certifications in Nutrition, Iridology, Reiki, International Aromatherapy through PIA, Master Practitioner of Neuro-Linguistic Programming (NLP), Master Practitioner of Hypnotherapy, PhD in Psychoneurology & Integrated Medicine, Anthony Robbins Digital Delivery Event Leader and as a Personal Trainer. Marcella Vonn is an inspirational mentor and coach in manifesting and teaching how to achieve one's divine purpose with grace and ease and fun.

You're quite outstanding in many ways to say the least. Why don't you give our audience that are listening, because I know many people have been excited to hear from you and to hear more about oils and how they can be used to enrich self-care and people's lives. Talk to us about your history and how you got involved with Young Living Oils and oils in general.

Vonn: Well thank you Robyn. It's amazing how I got involved in the world of aromatherapy and essential oils. It goes back to about 26-27 years ago, when no one in the world knew what an essential oil or aromatherapy was, at least here in the U.S. They were considered snake oils and anyone that was touting them around was considered a snake salesman, but how I got involved in this world of the smell and potent drops of plant essences is this.

I gave birth to a little girl October 16, 30 years ago and when she was inside of me, right before birth she had a bowel movement, which is called 'meconium', which is the first bowel movement a child has. She actually, through the stress of birthing, swallowed that bowel movement, so when she was born they suctioned her lungs for six and a half hours. I remember calling and asking, can I finally see my baby? That in itself is amazing because there's trauma just from that alone emotionally with abandonment issues, but basically it was touch and go for my baby.

We stayed in the hospital and she had a difficult time breathing. That never really got any better and at seven months of age she actually died in my husband's arms. We were rushed to the hospital where they resuscitated her back twice and we lived in ICU for about 12 days. My husband, Jim, and I believe that God gave her back to us. We had lots of complications. She didn't talk until she was almost three and the doctors and people of great authority in my life at the time, told me I would have to institutionalize her.

This is amazing too, because here in the U.S. we do so much with labeling and words. In Japan they have no word for retarded in their language and they have no retarded people, so I'm amazed at what we do with labels in this country. Robyn, this put me on a path of searching for everything and anything I could do to make a difference for my daughter. I refused to institutionalize her. I went back to school for nutrition and started playing in that arena.

What makes the story somewhat interesting is that I'm married to a man that was a Burger King franchisee. We had 24 restaurants and for the last 45 years my husband has been involved in the fast food business. He just retired December 1 of last year. Upon going back to school I really started to look at everything that could make a difference and this is where it gets interesting with the them of our call today, with Pay It Forward. It's fascinating when you have friends and family around you that know you're searching for something and everyone that knew I was on this path started to come to me and share things they thought would make a difference for Courtney.

That's how I got involved in the world of aromatherapy and essential oils. I was in China studying Chinese medicine and there was a woman there named Mary, and we became pretty good friends. She knew I was looking for anything and everything that would make a difference for my daughter's life. She lived in Salt Lake and when she got back to Salt Lake she'd gone to a health fair where she met a man that had these little bottles of essential oils with handwritten labels. She called me and said Vonn, I think this thing called essential oils and aromatherapy will make a difference for Courtney.

I said I don't know anything about it. She said we can explore this together and that opened up a whole new world for me. These little essences of oils and I started putting them on Courtney's feet and let her smell them before she went to school and before a particular subject. Literally, the teachers started seeing a difference. Other parents started seeing a difference in Courtney with her behavior and learning. It opened up the door for me. Then I started inviting people to my home and gave them a little bottle of oil to smell and put on their body and it started to make a difference in people's lives. It was never about money. It was never about a business, it was just about seeing if we could add value and makes a difference. I was looking at everything possible. You name it, I know about it and so much of what's out there today is just marketing and hype.

Education has been very important to me I've gone back to school. I've actually written five books and it's really about looking to see if something has some credibility and if it's authentic and can make a difference. Today the world of essential oils and aromatherapy is a science that's coming to fruition. We're in hospitals all over the world. There are about 24 oils that create an environment for no staff or MRSA, which is really big. I will tell you today in a hospital or nursing home or any type of facility where you're meeting lots of people, that's probably one of our biggest fears, is a staff infection.

Robyn: Can you talk about what the top three oils are?

Vonn: The number one oil that creates an environment for no staff is called lemongrass. Basically, the safest place to put essential oils is the bottom of your feet. There are three places on the human body that we tell people you should never put oil… your eyes, because obviously that could affect your vision. We never want to see people pour oils into their ears but basically the whole body is on the ear lobe. I'm talking to an acupuncturist, so you know the whole body the ear if you turn it sideways looks like an embryo. So you can actually work with the whole body just by massaging the ears.

It is amazing. Then we have this place that everyone has all over the world and they call it different things. I call it 'happy land', so you want to be careful with happy land with essential oils. The reason why I share that with you is because the feet are the safest place to put essential oils, but lemongrass can be hot oil. The safest place to put lemongrass would be on your feet and it has a zone of inhibition up to 83% that creates an environment for no staph or MRSA, which is phenomenal. I know one of your favorite oils that you use at your clinic is Thieves Oil is fabulous in creating an environment for no MRSA.

Robyn: We love it. In fact, for anyone who's listening, I know we have a lot of people who are in the health world. We use it, like I have several treatment rooms so we spray between patients. We also have a diffuser that we love that we have brewing clove right now, but we love it. It's so appropriate for anywhere; homes, certainly healthcare centers and it would be great if it were in hospitals. Can you imagine?

Vonn: Actually, essential oils of Young Living are in over 50 hospitals throughout the U.S.

Robyn: That's fantastic.

Vonn: In England they have certified aromatherapists in all of their hospitals, so it's becoming a mainstream tool just like many tools such as acupuncture, naturopath. There are so many tools in our toolbox of what we can do to bring balance into people's lives. The most fascinating thing about essential oils is there are over 300 in the world today, but about 100 that we can readily get our hands available on and the majority of those oils are antibacterial, antiviral and antifungal.

As a doctor, Robyn, you know that today most people coming to see you it's really not bacteria that we're so worried about. Everywhere I turn there's an antibacterial soap. We're flooded in the market with that, but what do we have for viruses? What do we have that really protects us from viruses that literally can go around the world within 24/48 hours? Essential oils create an environment where no viruses can live. That's what's so powerful about essential oils.

One drop of peppermint oil is equivalent to 26-28 cups of peppermint tea, that's how concentrated they are. So just to share with you how this made such a difference in my life is, when I started putting essential oils on my daughter and letting her smell them and we embodied the essential oils into our lifestyle, it started to make a difference for my daughter, to the degree that we never institutionalized her and she graduated from college with a degree. She's a beautiful young woman and is getting married in February.

It's been a fabulous journey for me. In the beginning I didn't know a lot about them and people could get overwhelmed with the world of aromatherapy, but if you took all the top aromatherapists in the world today and locked them up in a room and said you could only have one oil, the majority of those aromatherapists would take lavandula gustafolia and that oil is considered the mother of all oils. It's lavender oil and it's phenomenal for people suffering from stress. It's also wonderful for the skin.

Robyn: Just to go back to your amazing story Vonn, about your daughter being a mom myself. My son, we struggled for two years and here I was already in a full-time practice for 13 years, but he had a serious case of eczema and I've been using Young Living Oils from when I was pregnant with my first child for calming and different ones to help with the birthing process, that were put on my feet. My doula was the one who introduced me to oils.

Just to know, for all of you out there that have kids, when your kids get sick it's scary and you don't always want to rush your child off to the ER and just to have things on Saturdays and Sundays when you don't have help right away, but to know that you could have these oils at your home at any given time is nice. What you're talking about right now, viruses and bacteria, can you talk a little also about molds and the oils, because I know that's a big issue. I think one of my all time favorite oils is the Oregano oil.

Vonn: Oregano is very hot oil, so you want to be careful with that on the skin it's high in fenols, which is a constituent. You definitely want to dilute that oil for the skin, but there are three oils that no bacteria, virus or fungus can live in and one of those is Oregano. The others are cinnamon and thyme oils. Those are three hot oils and when you put them on the skin, but there's no virus, bacteria or fungus that can live in the presence of those three oils.

The fascinating thing about mold is if you've had a bathroom that's exposed to a lot of water or had any type of plumbing challenges where you've had water where it shouldn't be, we get mold. The only thing that I know up to a certain time that would get rid of mold was actually bleach, but the truth is that mold comes back with bleach and bleach is very much a carcinogen to our bodies. It's very harsh.

There's a doctor named Edward R Close, who has worked with the EPA. This is a fascinating story of how this happened, but he lives back in Missouri and I live in Arizona so I couldn't even relate to this story, but they would actually bleach the sides of their house for mold in the east. I couldn't believe it. This woman had run out of bleach and she took our Thieves cleaner, Young Living has a household cleaner that is made with the blend of thieves and on one section of the house she used this cleaner. She did the rest of the house and her husband was really upset, he went out and got more bleach but she'd finished up the job.

A year later she had mold everywhere where they used the bleach but none where she'd used the cleaner. So they called in the EPA and did all these experimentations. There's a video and a book on this, a breakthrough discovery of a non-toxic solution to toxic mold. People don't realize that with mold we get spurs and black mold will actually kill us, so it can really create havoc in the human body. There's some research out there that says mold is cancer. I question all of that. I don't think there's a magic bullet for all one thing, but there's actually a number of books out there saying that.

The Thieves blend creates an environment for no mold. So if you were to take that household cleaner and not dilute it and clean a bathroom where you had mold in the shower, clean it a couple times and you wouldn't get the mold back. It's amazing. We have a diffuser that we recommend you put it there and go through at least two bottles of Thieves oil, 15 mm and run them on a 24/7 and it's amazing how that creates that type of environment where mold can't live. So a diffuser will linger the air, 2100 to 2300 sq. ft. and if you would diffuse in a home or business 10 minutes a day or every other day, that fine molecular mist of the oils will linger in the air up to 72 hours.

It's a way to create a safe environment for our work and where we live, from being antibacterial, antiviral and antifungal. When someone gets a cold usually everyone gets it, because we're all exposed to that same bacteria and viruses, so a diffuser is a great way to create a safe environment. I have a lot of doctors that diffuse in their offices. They don't do it all day but in the morning before patients show up and at lunch. They don't make a big deal about it but they create an environment where it's safe.

Kevin: The Thieves cleaner is that a mixture of essential oils?

Vonn: Yes. It's an essential oil blend with eucalyptus, cinnamon and lemon and clove. It's a wonderful blend. The combination of this blend is fabulous how it invites such an environment but it also helps to boost our immune system. There isn't a time that I don't get on an airplane that I just take the Thieves oil and rub it on my feet. The thing is when we fly in an airplane people don't realize how exposed they are. If someone coughs and they have TB then everybody on that airplane has been exposed to TB. It is truly amazing and I feel it's one of the most dangerous places that we go all the time.

Robyn: I keep my Thieves spray in my purse all the time. Whether I'm in my car or in a plane since I travel a lot, that's what I do. I spray it on my hands and sniff it. People love sitting next to me because of it.

Vonn: It smells good.

Robyn: It smells great. Kevin, I don't know if you know that but we have all the Thieves cleaning products here too so we're set. This is flu season. The day after Thanksgiving I had three patients with major coughs and the other patients were like, I don't know if I want to be here, but I said just know that we do our best. We do everything possible. I never turn away a sick person that's what I do for a living. I say what I'm doing with you is I'm helping to boost your system because you don't worry about the sick person that's sitting next to you or across the way. If you get sick it's because of your weakened immune system.

Maybe you could share, since we're on this topic, about how you use oils for preventative medicine and keeping your immune system strong.

Vonn: The Thieves is definitely an oil I do to keep my immune system strong. Young Living has come out with a whole line of Thieves products, including a toothpaste and mouthwash.

Robyn: I have those too.

Vonn: I will tell you this. As a doctor, people don't realize that oral hygiene is everything to your health. If you lay out the blood vessels of the human body and you lay them end-to-end they will go around the globe of the earth at least one time. So if you have any infection in your mouth it's feeding your whole body, so oral hygiene is one of the biggest musts in creating a strong immune system. People don't really think about it so much like that either, but it's very strong.

Young Living has throat lozenges. Just using a great soap that's antibacterial, antiviral is good. The spray that we have from going to the grocery store and spraying it on the handles of the shopping carts. There are a lot of things we can do to help our health. One of those things is simply by getting a good night sleep and definitely all disease in the human body starts with dehydration, so we definitely have to hydrate our bodies.

But also we have to listen to our bodies. Most of us today poison ourselves over 30 times before we leave the house in the morning, just from all the commercial products we're using that are full of petrochemicals and toxins, thinking that we smell nice. My husband and I stopped wearing perfumes and colognes many years ago and just started wearing essential oils. Some people think we smell good and some think we stink, which is the same as it was with perfumes. Most of the perfumes out there today are made with toxins and it's amazing how so many people now are having a challenge.

If you work in an environment and someone comes in with a perfume that's made with petrol chemicals and poisons, how it affects everyone in that office because suddenly they have allergies and they can't tolerate. They're fatigued, they don't feel good and their nose is running. It's all because our bodies are exposed to so many toxins that we're in overload today.

Robyn: Exactly. We're exposed to 80k toxins at any given time and to know that you can have these essential oils with you at any time to protect yourself, because you never know. From indoors to being in your cars, which are toxic, so having that protection on your body when you wake up, is that what you recommend? When people wake up in the morning and take a shower is that a good time to put the oils on?

Vonn: That's a fabulous time. It's actually a fabulous time to even put the oils on while you're in the shower. We have bath gels and when you're wet or just drying off and you add essential oils to your skin, water dries essential oils deep into the skin, so it's fabulous to put them on after getting out of a shower in the morning.

Robyn: I know your travel schedule, you are amazing. You're literally around the globe a couple times and you never seem to be sick ever.

Vonn: No, I really take care of myself. There isn't a day that goes by where I don't put essential oils on my body, but it's like the simple things of life, getting a good nights sleep. I think attitude is the aroma of your heart. If your attitude stinks then your heart isn't in the right place. I think there are a lot of things that bring about health and what we do. Essential oils deliver 21-28% more oxygen uptake to the body, so if you're doing research in the world today about oxygen, we know that cancer can't live in an oxygen rich environment.

And, if our cells never lost the ability of oxygen then they would thrive, so we would live longer. So oxygen is a key component to the health of our body. This whole theme of this month of paying it forward, how do we do that? One of the things I'll share with you is when I became involved in Young Living I was basically looking at this selfishly for how it could make a difference for my daughter and at the time I had a girlfriend that lives not far from me. She called me after having been diagnosed with breast cancer.

They found a tumor on her left breast about the size of a half dollar and they recommended that she have a double mastectomy. This is like 16 years ago or more. They booked her for surgery and her surgery was like 3 ½ weeks away from when she came to see me. My background was a nutritionalist and we were talking about the diet and not being a medical doctor I couldn't advise her, but as her girlfriend I would go for a second opinion, because a double mastectomy was pretty drastic.

She went for a second opinion and they said the same thing and I called my friend, Mary, and said do we have any oils that make a difference with cancer? Mary said you know Vonn, there is a French encyclopedia book that's written by the French doctors and there are a couple oils in there that actually talk about cancer that are anti-tumoral and anti-cancerous. I said how do you use them? She said in the U.S. you couldn't take oils internally 20 years ago, whereas today you can if they're regulated by the government. There's a list called GRAS (Generally Regarded as Safe for Human Consumption). So there are oils that we can take internally and frankincense is one of those oils now, but frankincense oil, Boswellia Cartia was the oil that was listed in this aromatherapy medical encyclopedia.

Mary sent me all the information on it and my girlfriend came over and I said I'm not a doctor so I can't diagnose or prescribe, I can't even tell you what to do, but basically if this were me I would put this oil on my breast and in a diffuser. I told her that I would put a towel over my head and diffuse that oil about 10 minutes every morning and night where it was concentrated, where I could get it into my nose and breathe it in and into my lungs. She did that and she also put it in honey. The French would take oils internally and they would put them on bread and in honey. She did that and 2 ½ weeks later she couldn't feel the tumor at all. She came to me and I said you'll need to go back to your doctor.

She went back to the doctor and asks if they will run some tests and of course her doctor was quite furious with her and said even if you can't feel the tumor doesn't mean that it's not there and they were staying with the surgery. She was very emotional, she came home and talked to her husband who said what would it cost to run these tests maybe we'll just pay them ourselves? They went back to the doctor and ran the tests on their own, paying for it out of their own pocket and the tests came back that she'd been misdiagnosed. She never had to have the surgery.

That was the first year I had gotten involved in Young Living after making a difference for my daughter. That's a very close girlfriend still today. Talk about paying it forward, there isn't a day that goes by that takes my passion from traveling all over the world to tell people that essential oils can be just one more tool in their toolbox. There are lots of different things we can do in our lives, including acupuncture and the things that we do, and I don't take away from medicine either because there are times when we sometimes need that.

What I get passionate about is people knowing about all the different tools they have that can bring about balance and protect us in our life today. That's where my passion comes from and that's where it's all about paying it forward. There's a little saying that says *every great success is an accumulation of thousands of ordinary efforts that no one sees or appreciates.* I think that's what it is for us in everything that we do and even you as a doctor, the little things you say and do, we don't think anything of them we just keep doing them. I think that can make a big difference in people's lives.

Robyn: I love that statement.

Vonn: Ever since I met you and Kevin and had the opportunity to be with you at your clinic in Santa Fe, I have a sense that this is the stuff you do everyday. You're making a difference in so many people's lives everyday and you aren't being appreciated for some of the stuff you do or acknowledged for some of it, but you know that it's what makes your life and your practice successful. That's really what paying it forward is all about it's about being able to go to bed at night knowing that if it's your last day on the planet that you made a difference in someone's life.

Robyn: Absolutely. It rings so true for you too, Kevin, that when we were visioning the Self-Care Revolution™, we know what we do with our individual clients day in and day out, but when you think about it, like right now we have a global audience of thousands of people that are realizing that one of the most amazing pathways, this great gift that we have is a birthright to be your own best healthcare advocates. Just to have that great joy of taking care of yourself, what a difference.

Vonn: And I'm right in alignment with you Robyn, because I believe that essential oils are our birthright. They are the first plants on the earth. Plants and food will be our medicine today.

Robyn: Absolutely. When I met Gary Young, just to look into his face and hear him speak from his heart and his journey in creating this amazing opportunity for so many people, not only in the oils but also for all the people who work the business. These are just people in their homes getting this great gift out to their friends and families, which is the Pay It Forward that you're speaking about. But also, it's the science and dedication that this one man has put into producing the best possible product for all of us to use. Talk about paying it forward, he's done so much and just hearing of his travels I thought, talk about passion and commitment and to see what you've done in these 30 years Vonn is just awesome.

Vonn: Thank you. I'm gifting a *Yes, No Maybe*, it's the first book I wrote and it's basically on Chinese medicine. It's about eating in time, not necessarily what we eat but when we eat and how every organ of the body, all of us are cyclical, everything runs in cycles from our bio rhythms to our circadian rhythms to everything that we do. I'm gifting this book as a free gift. I was on CNN twice with this book. The reason for the title of the book is because everything in life, there are certain foods we can tolerate that maybe aren't the best foods we should be eating, yet we can get away with it, which is where the maybe comes in.

In life we basically will oftentimes eat so much of a certain food that we'll get sick of that food and then we won't eat that food anymore. People have experienced that with alcohol. It's fascinating with the human body to eating in time, that everything given in the right amount and right time can be beneficial for the human body or it can be a poison to the human body.

Kevin: We have that offer on our website at JoinTheSelfCareRevolution.com on Marcella's speaker page. Tell us your website where they can also get a hold of this.

Vonn: The link is on that and if they go to MVonn.com and say that they heard this on the Self-Care Revolution™ then we will follow up and get the book sent to them.

Robyn: What a wonderful gift. I have that book and for everyone listening, there's so much information in there and it's totally a Chinese medicine idea too that there are certain foods and maybe you can go into that Vonn, just mention what foods are best. You said that my chocolate habit and it's okay to have my dark chocolate in the morning.

Vonn: The thing is there really aren't any bad foods. We'll live in a world where I know there are people who are going to fight me on that from the GMO foods to the toxins and things out there, but basically there's poison in every food. There's arsenic in apples. There's cyanide in peaches. There's solenoid in potatoes. Every food has a poison in it. It's on a trace element that we need all of that for the body to work. I actually believe that through the periodic table we have all those elements in the body, even in trace elements.

The book is basically based on what flourishes and gives the planet energy. Our answer to that question would be the sun and if you look at the human body we're light beings. What gets the sun first thing in the morning is trees and things that grow on trees, which would be fruits and nuts. You need five things for every meal to be balanced, that's your protein, lipids, fats, carbohydrates, vitamins and minerals and water. Those are the things that you need in each meal so that it's balanced.

If we eat food when it's absorbing the energy of the planet, which first thing in the morning are things that grow on trees. Breakfast, the word itself is breaking a fast. So you want to eat foods that are easy in the morning, which are fruits and nuts will give you the lipids and proteins. I'm a big advocate for almonds, because they're fabulous and they're the king of all nuts. It's a hard nut so you need to soak it in water for like six hours so you can start breaking down the enzyme so it's easy to assimilate on the body.

→ So you eat nuts and fruit in the morning, easy meal.

→ Lunch is the biggest meal of the day. It is foods and what grows right above the ground, 4 inches to 4 feet above. That's your biggest meal of the day and should include meat, dairy and wheat.

→ Then foods at night would be those that grow under the ground, which would be potatoes, asparagus, eggs and fish. The nighttime foods all produce melatonin, serotonin and dopamine, so we wouldn't have the chemistry of all the antidepressants and things going on because food would actually bring our mind into balance.

We can get it through all the foods we eat, given that you eat them in the right times. The book is based on that and there's a chapter in the book on essential oils and how to use oils in time. There's a therapy chart which the whole book is based on, so if you have a respiratory or digestive issue, every hour to every two hours in a 24 hour cycle we actually give you a remedy to help bring the body into balance and it's all based on Chinese medicine.

Robyn: What a great gift. For all of those who are listening, you have this opportunity to go to Vonn's website at MVonn.com and she'll send it to you.

Kevin: I have lots of questions, many of which have been answered, so I appreciate Vonn sharing with us from her heart. She is definitely a true example of the Pay It Forward message and being of service in the world. We appreciate that. We were talking about the Thieves oil and I was impressed with how it came to be.

Vonn: Yes, it's a fascinating story and it's fascinating because Gary Young was introduced to essential oils in a cancer clinic down in Mexico in the early 80s. He had gone to Europe to study. Essential oils were more of a mainstream in Europe than they were in the U.S. So he had gone through the British archives, the library and he found two recipes that were written up in history and one was the story of this family of apothecary's who basically turned into thieves.

During the 17th Century bubonic plague, they went in and robbed the dead of their jewels and things they had. They were caught by the king and that's why the story is recorded in history. They used spices and oils on their body and they did not get sick, so it was written down and Gary came across that story and created the oil blend thieves. I believe out of all Young Living oils that it's one of the greatest things we could do to maintain a healthy and wonderful immune system.

It's like what Robyn said earlier, it actually comes down to it that that's all we have is our immune system. It's like what makes your immune system stronger than someone else's is how you're taking care of yourself and what you're putting in your body, what's coming out of your body and the environment in which you live. So there are certain things we can do that make such a major difference in our health and longevity.

Kevin: I know just seeing the line of oils that are available through Young Living, myself included, like you said earlier it can be a little overwhelming as to what to have in my medicine cabinet. What would you recommend as the top five self-care oils to have?

Vonn: That's a fabulous question. One of the things Young Living did is to create a basic starter kit with 10 oils. That's a fabulous way to get started. Before telling you about those 10 oils I will share with you that aromatherapy is pretty much known all over the world today, but not the quality of oils. The sad thing is that there are so many oils today on the market from little boutiques to galleries and health food stores that literally you go in and some of them smell good and some don't. Some cost from pennies up to hundreds of dollars, but the majority of those oils is something you'd never want to put on your skin, being that your skin is the largest organ of the body, let alone smell.

The last couple of years we've come out with vaccinations that we deliver through the nasal cavity, so it's amazing our sense of smell and how it affects our body, but there's so much junk out there today in the world of marketing and what somebody would call an essential oil of aromatherapy, it's really sad. Young Living is a company that's in over 100 different countries around the world and they're the only company of oils that I would actually take internally in my body or even put on my skin.

There at your clinic in New Mexico, you can pick up the oils but it's important that we're talking about a good quality product that we're diffusing in our homes or taking into our bodies or putting onto our skin. That start kit that Young Living has come out with, when I look at the top aromatherapists in the world that only use 10 oils in everything they do, that's basically where we went in taking out the overwhelm for people in the world of aromatherapy and finding 10 oils that could make a difference in your life. Those oils, like lavender, it's the number one oil for anything to do with the skin and anybody that's stressed or has a lot of anxiety, putting lavender on the bottom of your feet can make all the difference in the world.

You go into the department stores and look at cleaning supplies and everything smells of lemon. Your bath products all smell of lavender. Lavender is calming for the body. Going back to lemon in the cleaning products, lemon is a degreaser, but the lemon oil is very different than lemon juice. When you go to a nice restaurant they put a slice of lemon in your water, the lemon oil comes from the rind and it will purify your water. Peppermint oils is in the kit and Kevin, that's the number one oil for digestive challenges.

People that don't feel good… when you go to a nice restaurant they have a great thought in giving you a peppermint mint after you've eaten your meal. There's probably no therapeutic quality in the candy they're giving you even though the thought was great, because peppermint is fabulous for any type of digestive issues. In a small trial if I took peppermint oil and rubbed it on the bottom of their feet it would bring down a fever.

On a very hot day like we have here in Arizona and you're in Santa Fe, if I were to take one drop of peppermint and put it in my water it would bring down my body temperature and I carry it when I travel in case I get a little nauseas or motion sickness, just one drop on the tongue, fabulous.

Robyn: I want to interrupt just a quick minute. What you're sharing is touching upon an overriding theme of the Self-Care Revolution™ but it's all about returning to nature. Even when you talk about the lemon that comes from many restaurants, it's not necessarily organic and you don't know who's touched that thing but when you get that oil going into your water you know the purity of it. It's the same with peppermint, one that's laden with sugar as opposed to the actual peppermint oil, getting back to nature 100% from what the earth provides, there's nothing better and it's the ultimate self-care message. The cells want nature not all these extra toxins and pollutants added to it.

Vonn: Robyn that's the big point is it's all about self-care. It's like how do we really start taking care of ourselves on an individual basis everyday? One drop of oil can go a long way and one drop can be antibacterial, antiviral, anti-cancerous, anti-tumoral, it's amazing. Inflammation is the number one cause of all disease in the human body today and yet there's essential oils that bring down inflammation in the body. It's going back to nature and to looking at what we can do everyday. Most of us are putting stuff on our bodies that smell, but if we were to switch those over to essential oils it could be amazing what they could do for health.

Also, one of the offers that I have is to give people the small EDR and essential desk reference, where they can look up and get educated on how to actually use essential oils and aromatherapy. I'm a real believer that in self-care we have to educate ourselves. It's about us taking responsibility for our health and what we do and not pointing the finger to someone else. That's the biggest step we have to deal with in self-care is how do we actually start to really take care of ourselves, in a way where we're getting results and we're feeling better.

Kevin: Absolutely and this is on your speaker page of our website, the EDR. For anyone listening to the call right now who's excited about this particular product line and what Vonn is sharing with us, click on it and receive the desk reference and get started on this amazing path of healing. It is an incredible gift that you're sharing with us today.

Vonn: If anyone out there listening to this that's using essential oils and it may not be Young Living, please feel free to give me a call and let's talk to really look and see. One of the first things I tell people is to read the label on the bottle. If it says do not eat or take internally then you have to know right there you have a problem with that product.

Kevin: Right.

Robyn: So this is probably a good time to mention if people want to make the investment and buy them on their own, I just want to mention too that the Self-Care Revolution™ if you go to the shop section, we only have six different things that we are supporting. The Berry Breeze, which is something, you put in your refrigerator to enliven and keep your produce alive for an extra two weeks. We also have the MRS mat that basically mimics nature to enliven and uplift the health of every cell in your body but you'll see Young Living oils there as well, so we don't have hundreds of things we only have a few things that we're behind 100% that are in line with the self-care message that is about nature.

Could you explain to people listening that might want to go to make this investment themselves so they have their own oils at home?

Vonn: That's great but I also want to mention that in all the world out there with network marketing companies they come and go, whereas Young Living has been around for over 20 years and to share with you, we are a product-driven company. When you come to Young Living you aren't going to see the hype of the whole network marketing arena, 83% of our company is just product users. So I explain to people that we're basically just like Costco, you come in to the company as a member and you have an opportunity to buy retail or you can buy wholesale, but if you choose to become a member then there's this premier kit that gives you 10 oils for $150 plus a diffuser.

It's a great value and it has a money back guarantee with it, where even if you go through all the oils and products within 60 days and you don't feel there's value, I will write you a check and give you all your money back for it. So 83% of our company is product users, which again is how we Pay It Forward. We're in a place of seeing how we can start to make a difference on this planet and we start with one person at a time, us taking care of us first.

Kevin: That's so true and such a great message.

Vonn: So your question as to which oils they get for their homes...

Robyn: Maybe talk about the upgrade bonus you have here, the essential program.

Vonn: If someone does choose to get involved in Young Living and go through the websites, we will personally reach out to you no matter where you are in the world to connect with you, as well as educate you to the product that you'd be getting and what you would do with them. That's the whole thing about self-care. Again, if you don't know what you have or how to use it it's not going to do you any good, so education is big for our company. It's a big piece for me as well, because when I got involved in these products 25 years ago it was important that I knew how to use them to make a difference for myself and my daughter.

The information is there. The essential rewards program is one where if you choose to have these products in your life than we're going to give you every type of bonus and tool that we can to make your life easier. We have a website that educates you to the products and how to use them, what to do and how to share them with people. You'll get that free, a customized website for the essential rewards program. Those are all bonuses that we're offering.

Kevin: It's so important and I think this product and the way you're sharing it is a perfect connection to Pay It Forward. I've been exposed to these oils for probably 15 years myself and I often run into people and this is how they deliver this message. I had a bad ear infection and someone said if you'd just drop a little of that Thieves in there in a few hours the pain in the ear will subside and it did, so they gave the bottle of oil to me. It's a powerful thing to be able to do for people, to share these products and this message, as well as the education, which is an important piece.

Vonn: The genius behind Bill Gates, Warren Buffet and every other mega success was their ability to work through other people to achieve their grand vision. I know the grand vision, Kevin and Robyn, is self-care and what that looks like all over the world. It's amazing how they were masters at getting people to work towards a common goal, while achieving their personal goals. Again, self-care is what it's all coming down to. We're living in a world today, from Obama Care and everything that's happening out there, where we really need to take responsibility for keeping our immune system strong today and how we can do that.

I think how we start doing that is starting to look at the environment, which we live in. That's why I'm a big advocate that every home should have a diffuser to diffuse the oils. They discovered that the most toxic environment in which we go to everyday is our homes. It's funny how fire retardant is one of the most toxic things and it's on our furniture, our clothes and mattresses, so it's affecting our health every day. What are we doing about these things? Essential oils breaks down those petrol chemicals, so it's amazing how just diffusing an oil can make such a major difference.

I came across some information the other day that was fascinating, in that here in the U.S. we spend $15 billion on ice cream yearly. We spend $45 billion on pet food. We spend $61 billion on weight loss products and $160 billion on skin care. I'm like wow, that is an amazing amount of money and yet, where is it taking us? Is it making a difference in our lives right now? I'm thinking one little drop of oil can make such difference in people's lives, so for me paying it forward is about educating people to the world of aromatherapy and essential oils.

Robyn: I love that you're talking about this. In my practice I have essential oils in each room, but so many people as we know, we're stressed out beyond belief so when people lie on my table I'll add lavender and sometimes peppermint if someone has a headache and I love thieves, I use that a lot because some of these people are grieving and there's a lot to grieve about in today's world. I find that people get centered. It's amazing how one drop can center a person.

I carry lavender and thieves all the time in my purse and it's just so nice, whether I'm at a gathering or whatever, where I can pull it out and share it with somebody. So it's nice that it doesn't have to be a medical thing, because we can share in everyday life with our friends and family. Our kids are growing up in a much different world, I'm 48 with a 12 and 14 year old, and they're exposed to so many more toxins than I was and we have a diffuser at home also. It's just another way that I keep my kids healthy. We do use Oregano oil straight, I hope that's okay, on the feet at night.

Vonn: Yes.

Robyn: Just to have that sense of, oh my gosh, I always have something 24/7 that I can use for my own health and immune system, as well as to share with someone else.

Vonn: The 10 oils that Young Living starts you with, I could actually do a redo on your whole medicine cabinet for that. I'm always telling people, why are there never any good side effects from all the medical drugs today? Just once I'd like to read a medication bottle that says it may cause extreme sexiness.

Robyn: I like that.

Kevin: If you're finding this interview anywhere other than our website it's JoinTheSelfCareRevolution.com and if you have any questions for us or Vonn, email us at info@jointheselfcarerevolution.com.

Robyn: If you listen to this replay Pay It Forward. In fact, we'll keep this live longer because we want to get this message out to thousands of people. The message of the Self-Care Revolution™ the mission is to impact a billion people with this message, being your own self-help care advocate, which is one of the greatest privileges we each have and adding the oils into your daily life is a perfect way to do that everyday.

Vonn: I agree. One of the easiest ways to find me is to go to MVonn.com.

Kevin: You started the list of 10, so let's see if we can finish that up in our last few minutes.

Vonn: We have a blend called peace and calming. Gary formulated this to get children off of Ritalin. Even hyper active dogs, simply rub this in their ears and it makes all the difference in the world. There's a blend in the 10 oils called purification, which was a blend that will stop any itching on the body. It will create an environment to protect you from mosquitoes and those no-see em' bugs. It also will neutralize smells from dog odors to cooking fish in your kitchen to cigarette smoke. The blend of thieves that you get in the kit and frankincense oil is also in the kit.

There's peppermint and how it's a wonderful oil for digestion. Lemon is also in there and Gary put a blend called joy oil in there, which has one of the most expensive oils in the world in it and that is Rose oil. It's a wonderful perfume blend. They say people cannot be depressed smelling roses, that this oil of Rose is the highest frequency plants when they measure frequencies on all plants on the planet. I think that's fascinating because the saints in churches resonate with the smell of roses. I think that's it.

Robyn: I want to say once more that your book offer is amazing. We've had speakers offer a chapter or two, but you're shipping an entire physical book to each person that requests it. That is beyond generous. I have the book and I love it. Plus, being in your presence and seeing how you share this information with everyone you know, it's great. We've been using this in our home and it's fabulous. For me as a Doctor of Oriental Medicine, 21 years later, to continue to learn and I've learned from reading your book. It is wonderful.

Thank you for what you're doing in the world and sharing your great gift and taking this out to so many different groups. I love your passion. You've been doing this for nearly 30 years and you're still going at it 100%, so thank you for sharing with our great audience of self-care revolutionaries so much information.

Vonn: Thank you Robyn and Kevin for the opportunity. I think that's what self-care is all about is actually paying it forward. When we find something that makes a phenomenal difference in our life to share it with others, so thanks for this opportunity to share with you.

Robyn: Thank you.

[End of Interview]

DEBORAH KOPPEL MITCHELL

ConsciousMeme.com | One of the Founders of The Conscious Meme, contributing-author of the books *"From Inspiration to Realization"* and *"Conscious Choices: An Evolutionary Women's Guide to Life"*

THE CONSCIOUS MEME

[These statements have not been evaluated by the Food and Drug Administration. The information on this audiocast is not intended to diagnose, treat, cure, or prevent any disease.]

Robyn: Hello everyone and welcome to month 12 of the Self-Care Revolution™, what a year it's been. What a month it's been. Kevin, wouldn't you say this Pay It Forward month has been, talk about a revolutionary subject. I feel like it's changed my life. Everyday I'm thinking about this Pay It Forward idea and sharing all the wealth of information that we've learned in these 12 months with so many people and sharing the gift of life in this holiday season.

We have a wonderful speaker today, Deborah Koppel Mitchell, hello, how are you?

Deborah: Hello, I'm so glad to be here.

Robyn: Welcome. For everyone listening for the very first time, my name is Robyn Benson. I'm a Doctor of Oriental Medicine and the Founder of Santa Fe Soul Health and Healing Center, and a self-care revolutionary in a big way. It's been a joy listening to the incredible jewels of information and knowledge that each and every one of our speakers has shared since month one, where we started out with thoughts and food as medicine.

Today I'm joined with my fabulous co-host.

Kevin: Hi, I'm Kevin Snow and what an incredible journey it has been this year and what a great month and great way to finish up this year, this Pay It Forward message again with amazing gratitude to you, Robyn, for spearheading this revolution and the incredible people that have been part of this revolution this year to include: speakers, contributors and co-hosts. Thanks Harmony for being there today. It's been an incredible journey and I'm truly grateful.

Robyn: Kevin, we know you have to leave but thank you for being here for the introduction of our sweet speaker, Deborah Mitchell.

Harmony: Thanks Kevin. I'm Harmony West. I'm a family health and wellness educator at Santa Fe Soul Health and Healing Center. I'm glad to be here at the tail end of 2013 in the Pay It Forward month.

Robyn: So Deborah, again welcome and for everyone, Deborah is a messenger and publisher of conscious raising publications and movements. She is a contributing author of, *From Inspiration to Realization and Conscious Choices*, an evolutionary women's guide to life. Deborah is the modern day Pollyanna, re-defining what it means to be a "Pollyanna" and is Founder of the Conscious Meme network. It's so great to have you with us, Deborah. We have a cool topic that I think many people don't even know what it meme means.

Deborah: A lot of people even see meme written down and say me-me, so I have people ask me all the time what a me-me is.

Robyn: Why don't you give us a little background of how you got to be known as the Pollyanna or how this content of work became important to you and this whole meme movement? Give us some background about you and all the fabulous work you're doing.

Deborah: Thank you. I started being a part of the women's spirituality movement back in 98'. I started doing women's circles, which I facilitated for 14 years, which led into starting a grassroots magazine publication called *'The Spheres'*; Women's Circles Publication which transitioned into a sphere circle, the Yen Yang Magazine for women and men and then transitioned into being an online magazine and now, just this week we launched the Meme Messenger E-zine. This is all about shining a light on what elevates our lives and spreading ideas that matter, which brings me to the meme, if you'd like me to let the listeners know what a meme is.

It seems, Robyn, like you are a person who really just got it as soon as you heard about it. My founding partner, Christie Revelus, and, I–we were two of those people. We heard the word meme, Christie was using it in the context of describing something and she said and that hasn't been memed yet. At the time I didn't know what the word meme meant, I couldn't define it, but it was like the lights went off. I knew in the context of what she was saying what it meant. I got almost like a wave; a feeling and I knew it was big and that it was important.

We got very excited about looking up what the definition of meme was. Christie is a coach and she's used the word before after hearing it and that week she had that book fall off her shelf called *Virus of the Mind*; The New Science of the Meme, written by

Richard Brody which was written in the 90s. When we looked up the definition of meme, it said it was an unconscious cultural virus, a thought, an idea or behavior, anything that goes mainstream or viral and the thing that stood out to us was that it was unconscious.

We thought what would happen if we came up with the phrase conscious meme and brought about meme awareness, awareness of the things that run us unconsciously and also to encourage the formation of what we're calling conscious memes, which are for the highest good of all. It's creating trends, ideas and behaviors that actually have a positive effect on all. We also found that the word meme was actually coined by Richard Dawkins in 1976. He was a British evolutionary biologist and he coined it in his book called *The Selfish Gene*.

So we just started creating a movement which we started, especially on Facebook, call the Conscious Meme Movement and since then, Robyn, like so many things, like when you decide you're going to buy a car and you're thinking about it so you start seeing that particular car everywhere. The word meme seems like it's popping up everywhere. We're a part of meme-ing the word meme and I'd really love to share with you and all the listeners why we should even care about what a meme is, like why am I so excited? In Richard Brody's book, one of the statements he made that really stood out was that meme awareness could improve the qualities of our lives. That hit us like a wave and made us realize that we were really onto something.

Harmony: Talk more about that and what you're onto.

Deborah: The thing is that's fun on a small scale is in starting our movement and talking to friends, people are becoming more aware of the memes that are in our lives and the things that are running us unconsciously and starting to ask questions. It's very important to be aware and start asking questions of, what's influencing me that I'm not aware of and what is my truth here, what is real? You start noticing on many levels of our culture, all the memes that are out there as far as branding things, health, our family influences, prejudices and things that we call negative memes or what we're calling conscious memes.

Regarding negative memes, an example would be prejudice, people having fear-based ideas like even about we're in a full moon right now so some people get nervous around a full moon. Why is that? Because people have said others get crazy when it's a full moon. Now it seems like things are shifting because people are becoming more conscious of how their thoughts and behaviors affect everything. They are choosing to focus on the more positive aspects of things, like the full moon being a time to set your intentions, to take time to focus and have rituals and create a more sacred environment and things like that.

Robyn: Maybe you could speak about the meme movements that are out there right now, like the Pay It Forward.

Deborah: There are organizations that would like to bring us back to conscious memes that are happening that are phrases or ideas such as, your whole Pay It Forward. That became a conscious meme that was triggered from a film of the same name. How about random acts of kindness. People relate when they hear that phrase now. The law of attraction, which the film The Secret, which that film became meme. It went viral. It went mainstream and now whenever you say someone was in The Secret, most of us in our society know what that was. The people that were in The Secret, one of their biggest promotions when they're out speaking in the world is that they'll say, I was in The Secret.

How about the whole idea of being of service, that it seems like that really became more mainstream after President Obama and Michelle put a call out to our country to start being of more service. There are polls and studies that show that there was a huge increase, which continues as people continue being more of service. Some of the organizations out there that we're really excited about and on our website, TheConsciousMemeNetwork.com, we have a resources page that's filled with books and organizations and people that are making a positive impact on the world, which is their intention with everything they're doing.

We have people like AGE Nation, which some friends of ours launched and it's all about creating solutions, education and inspiring people to age consciously and make good decisions for the rest of their lives. I know they were on your show.

Robyn: They were, we loved our interview with them in month 10, Be Fabulous at Any Age.

Deborah: Yes, Sedena and George Cappannelli, dear friends of ours and they're starting to meme. When people see a film that is on people in the second half of life and we're sitting there, friends will say that's a real AGE Nation film. Organizations like Barbara Marks Hubbards Foundation for Conscious Evolution, bringing awareness and knowledge for transitioning during our evolutionary times and consciousness. Barbara's been memed as a public figure. Oprah is memed, along with

Oprah's Super Soul Sunday. All of these are considered conscious memes. As soon as it becomes something that goes mainstream or viral, and YouTube is a wonderful example of creating memes that can either be disgusting or raising our consciousness.

Whole films have been on YouTube and gone meme, like The Secret and the Thrive movement film.

Robyn: Proctor was also one of our speakers.

Deborah: Yes, Proctor and Kimberly Gamble, everything they're doing and putting out there with their blogs. They're always highlighting some of the actual positive things that are happening in the world. They had a posting recently showing throughout the country where people are rebelling that some of the enforcers are actually starting a trend where they're becoming gentler and sympathetic to causes and not attacking people. It's a movement. We need to hear about these positive things that are happening, because one of the big things that one of the big conscious memes that's out there now is on what we focus expands. We've all been hearing that it goes with the law of attraction.

So, it's our intention with the conscious meme movement to start shining a light on the things out there that are going on. There's so much happening that's of a positive nature and yet, still on the news and in most media everything is very negative and fear-based and sensationalized news. It's so important for us all to become more and more aware that we are the ones that create these mind viruses, these cultural viruses. If we start focusing on creating things that are for the higher good of all concerned, that will become the main focus, hopefully of the news of our world. That is what changes the quality of our lives and improves the quality as well.

Robyn: It's so great how you're sharing this huge way of looking at what a meme is and the power of these memes, the shifts that happen because of them. Even with the Self-Care Revolution™, our tagline is, self-care is the truth healthcare. That is our meme. That is our virus that we want to spread out to every single person's soul that each and every one of us has this incredible innate ability to take care of ourselves and we're designed to be well.

The more this spreads and this ripple of change that's already happening, the amount of people's lives that are not only going to be saved but also our mission to help people not only reverse but to prevent disease from happening in the first place. It's a massive meme and a lot of people ask why we're doing a 12-month program. Why is this series going on? It's because this is a true movement. If we just did, okay we're going to do the Self-Care Revolution™ for six weeks with 25 speakers; we didn't feel strongly that the meme, the impact of what's being created with this revolution would have the reach that it's had. We are also going strong in 2014 as well. We have a live event called the Self-Care Lifestyle Bliss event. This will be our second annual event.

Deborah: That's fantastic, and the fact that members of the Self-Care Revolution™ can continue to access the interviews, that creates the ripple effect because all over the place at different times and phases of time, people are re-listening and hearing these positive life enhancing messages. It's very important.

Robyn: We're also creating a book for every single month. Every module and theme has a book; the first has 11 speakers from month one. So Pay It Forward month with you Deborah we'll have your interview along with the six other speakers. I also wanted to mention that we're interviewing Charley Johnson, who started a global Pay It Forward movement. We're so excited to interview him. So, when you start talking about this meme message and how you've taken it from the book and now it's a movement, I was like yum, I so get it.

Deborah: Thank you. Another phrase that popped out at us in Richard Brody's book *Virus of the Mind; The New Science of the Meme*, was at the end of the book he called out to all of us to become meme ambassadors. We changed the phrase to meme emissaries, because we feel like we have a mission to spread this awareness and meme it. I've always been against labeling things and yet, when I heard the word meme, which can actually stand for so many things, because as we said before a thought, behavior or trend and idea, things that go mainstream why couldn't we just say that?

To have an actual word for it that you can carry with you in your awareness as you move through your life, which creates more consciousness around what it is that we're doing that we want to have other people emulate. That's where we came up with one of our moniker's which is 'you are it'. Memeing that phrase, you are it, you're the one. Each of us are the one, just like hearing that beautiful phrase, we're the ones we've been waiting for. You are it is like a piece of that. We're the ones, each of us, that can have an affect on everything in our lives. So if we start carrying that consciousness as we move through our lives we are having a beautiful ripple effect on everything.

That includes the spheres that are spinning in the universe, if we can just walk around and feel that fullness, connectedness and oneness when we think about conscious memes and who we want to be in the world and how we want to affect the world, that can affect our health and future and future generations.

Harmony: I love this and feel I resonate so much with your message. I think there may be those in the unconscious culture that would call you a Pollyanna.

Deborah: Yes, and you know what I say to that? I say thank you for calling me a Pollyanna.

Harmony: Talk about that, because that word Pollyanna doesn't have such bright cheery connotations my dear.

Deborah: That too is being changed by people like me, the modern day Pollyanna and people like Abraham Hicks who are out there telling people that they should be more Pollyanna. If someone calls him a Pollyanna they should say thank you, because that all comes back to the law of attraction. I would love to share how I was ignited around branding myself the modern day Pollyanna. It was back when The Secret first came out, I remember driving in my car and thinking about how it seemed like, with the law of attraction and people becoming more aware of how our thoughts create our reality and how important it is to think more positively and to have a higher vibration, that it seemed like the world was finally catching up with us Pollyanna's.

I had been teased about being a Pollyanna all my life. I was told I smiled too much. I was told I was too positive or I'd always find the good in everything. When Eleanor Porter wrote the book *Pollyanna* back in 1913, the main character was a young girl who had a positive attitude and outlook that infected an entire community positively. I don't know how or when but at some point in our culture, Pollyanna became memed as a negative connotation and in fact, it became a noun in the dictionary and is defined as a person who is positive to a fault.

Now you hear all sorts of people doing speeches throughout our lives saying, I don't mean to sound Pollyanna around this or I don't want to be thought of as a Pollyanna, but really because there has been a shift luckily and you hear more, and in fact, so many of your speakers for Self-Care Revolution™ their message is about the importance of our thoughts creating our reality and what kinds of vibrations we're carrying in our lives.

One of the things that I really want to bring an awareness around is changing the idea that a Pollyanna is a person who only sees the world through rose-colored glasses. It's really not about that it's more of what I said before about carrying a high vibration, which can be having compassion or patience and those two qualities for ourselves and learning to have an overview and seeing the big picture. Those things create a high vibration that affects everything. I really appreciate you doing the Self-Care Revolution™ and having so many of your wonderful speakers on whose message is exactly that, it's telling us the importance of having that higher vibration and positivity in the world.

Harmony: That's beautiful.

Robyn: I love that word, the power of positivity. I could just tell all the listeners that to this day you're vibrant Deborah and I love your positivity. I think it's fantastic that you didn't let that diminish your brilliance and your great message to so many. As we explored in month three, transmuting trauma and how many people, just by being labeled by something early on in life, how much that shut down their light. Thank you for being the bright light that you are in the world.

Deborah: Thank you. I would also like to share another piece of the higher vibration, which can be compassion. I've had to learn to walk my talk recently. I've been going through the grieving process around the passing of my dear brother, Daniel, back in May. I've never been through the grieving process and I feel like I have so much more compassion for people who are grieving. One of the things I had to hold for myself because I found this critical voice creeping in and telling me, hey you're not walking your talk because you're feeling so low or you're depressed or you're crying when someone asks how you are.

I had to really walk my talk around that compassion towards self and allowing for whatever may feel less than positive to actually move through me so I could come out the other side. That is definitely a part of positivity is allowing for things that look less than perfect or less than positive or don't feel good. Sometimes it's really about getting in that compassionate surrendered, allowing space of delving as deep as you need to go, so you can come out the other side.

Harmony: I think a lot of people think that being positive is putting a bright shiny face on all the time no matter what and that that's not true at all. What you're talking about is being authentic and being real with what it is you're experiencing.

Deborah: Yes and that authenticity touches everyone. I used to experience that in the circles that I did and that I know you do as well, Harmony. You really relate and know what I'm talking about when you experience someone sharing and going into story or if they get up on what feels like a soapbox where they're trying to teach you. Or, when someone is being totally authentic, even allowing themselves to cry or to laugh hysterically and it's authentic, you can feel that whole container and circle pull in and become energized. You can feel the energy being depleted by just being talked at.

Harmony: I'm wondering if so many of the unconscious memes that infiltrate our society helping us not to be our authentic selves. What you're talking about is going to the human condition of feelings and allowing them to be real and having it be a way that connects us as opposed to separating us.

Deborah: Yes, thank you for that. That brings me back to what I brought up before about becoming more aware of the things that run us unconsciously and also, starting to ask questions of, wait a minute is this really my truth and how I'm feeling? Is this how I'm feeling or am I feeling this way because I think I'm supposed to? Am I looking at this or this person or situation this way because I think I'm supposed to because it's been memed that way?

Harmony: Do you think there are a lot of us that are practicing this conscious memeing and is there enough of us to make a difference?

Deborah: It's interesting, when you said that I actually got goose bumps, because I was thinking about shows like Super Soul Sunday. My mom, who is homebound at 86, watches Super Soul Sunday every week and it totally uplifts her. That show has gone mainstream and Oprah features ongoing persons, thought leaders and inspirational people of our times, getting these messages out there mainstream. I think Dr. Oz has done that with his show as well, getting people like my parents, my dad and his wife who are a little more skeptical around some of the alternative health messages and modalities.

Thanks to Dr. Oz they're now telling me some of these things. I love it. Speaking of health, I wanted to bring up that Santa Fe Soul and Self-Care Revolution™ also has a focus on health and to start noticing some of the health memes that are out there. If you think about when everyone started running. I'm a runner have you run today, everybody was a runner and then this whole generation of people started having to have knee replacements and injuries. Now it seems like the new health exercise meme has geared more towards more gentle exercise like yoga, Pilates and things like that.

If you think about, have you noticed how much people are saying they're going gluten-free? We have so many out of town guests and I almost always have to send a questionnaire before they arrive regarding any special dietary needs. Almost everyone nowadays is gluten-free where before when people went gluten-free it seems like such a rare thing and you couldn't find hardly anything gluten-free in the grocery store or restaurants. Now you can go out and there are gluten-free items on menus and the grocery store is packed with gluten-free things. That's a meme, because it's for good health.

Robyn: Going from running being such a big thing to oh, I've put that aside. I'm like marathon running, what was I doing for all those years. I can do burst fit training for 20 minutes and get more from a workout and better overall health for my body on a cellular level than running an hour a day. We devoted an entire month to the theme of exercise is medicine, to get all the best memes out there from our incredible speakers. That's part of why we're getting these Self-Care Revolution™ books out there for each meme themes, to spread the good news and help people reclaim their health and to feel the vitality we all crave.

Deborah: A fun and energizing thought to me from our talk today is just thinking how even if just a few people that we've reached start noticing the memes that are in their lives and what a meme is and what isn't, start using the word and start educating other people on it and becoming more aware of wanting to create things that could go viral that are actually positive and could be for a higher good, then we've really done our job here today.

Harmony: It seems, Deborah, like so many of the unconscious memes are really money-driven and that what you're talking about are conscious means that are heart-driven, humanity-driven and are ways of connecting and uplifting and loving on all of us.

Deborah: Yes and the other side of that is if we can start moving through our lives noticing things that have gone mainstream that aren't for elevating us all, that are those dark memes, which Richard Brody talks about in his book, that's very important too. It's important for us to have the awareness of things that aren't working in our lives anymore and shifting those things. I believe that we have seen much in our society like we talked about before, of some of the programs that are so popular now that are out there and actually uplifting.

Remember, when all of a sudden we had all these reality shows that were so low vibration, which there are still quite a few of, but there are also some reality shows on now that before the networks probably thought wouldn't work because they were too positive which are working now. The Long Island Medium, I've watched a few of those shows and it's opened a lot of people's minds. Then there's Undercover Boss, which sounds so strange, but those are also moving. You can see someone make a huge leap into the type of person they are, start helping people and getting a grip on what's happening and caring. It's shifting and that's very encouraging.

Harmony: I don't watch much TV but I know over the course of my life I remember being a teenager doing yoga and people thinking that was the strangest thing on the planet and now who doesn't know what yoga is. Or, discovering natural foods when I was a teen and now everyone is into natural foods.

Robyn: It's a movement.

Harmony: So give your conscious meme some time and it will take over the planet.

Deborah: You become aware of the conscious memes that are taking over the planet. One of the fun things… I consider myself as being a baby boomer… is seeing how we baby boomers have influenced society and how there have been some big shifts and the contrast of the things that haven't made the shift are being much more exposed.

Robyn: Absolutely. I love this whole idea of you are it. That is such a powerful message to every one of us. I love the idea of being meme-ful. You're going to help get that word out there, because the virus word isn't always the most exciting, but that's one of the best ways to describe it or that hundredth monkey effect, that ripple change effect, but for people to really choose this as part of a meaningful life is engaging in these memes that, as Harmony said, are from the heart.

Deborah: Yes and the hundredth monkey theory is something I don't know if everyone knows about and maybe if we have a minute, it's about showing how critical mass can have an effect and how some things happen organically from a behavior and the hundredth monkey theory the way I understand is that there was a study of monkeys on one side of the planet and they were observed starting to wash potatoes or something and they had never done that before. Then suddenly they noticed that monkey's all over the planet were washing potatoes like it was a normal part of their behavior. That was a meme of behavior that happened amongst monkeys.

The same thing we have found with people, that type of the spreading of behaviors which is why again, the awareness of what we're doing and our intention behind what we're doing is critically important for the critical masses.

Harmony: I think part of the value of that story too is that the way the potato washing started was that one monkey, one person taught another who taught another who taught another and when there was really critical mass reached, there didn't have to be any direct teaching. It was in the cosmos, in the air and we're hoping that that's happening with the Self-Care Revolution™.

Deborah: Yes, just getting the phrase Pay It Forward out there again, that creates that positive ripple effect. I'm reminded just hearing it, of what I want to do that could be a Pay It Forward for something that was done for me that was kind or maybe nothing was done for me kind and I want to be the one to start the Pay It Forward movement.

Harmony: I spend so much time with children and see that they naturally do that. I was in a circle of girls yesterday and we were talking about something that felt really good throughout the day, something you wanted to share and it was beautiful to watch as one girl would share which would ignite something in someone else and then someone who just shared would say wait, I want to tell you something too. It was all of us focusing on ways that we supported other people or that people supported us. So you could see where it's all contagious.

Deborah: That's where being in circle or doing anything with others that is of a higher nature or sacred, creates that ripple affect because now those girls as they're moving about in their lives will be thinking about what could I share and they'll affect another and another. I love that about human beings.

Robyn: You talk about circles, why don't you share about *The Millionth Circle*.

Harmony: You're in the circle movement also and Jane Bolden who brought the Million Circle, talks about the hundredth monkey.

Deborah: Exactly. She was one of the first times I had ever heard of that story.

Harmony: I thought about that a number of times as we've been talking, the whole idea of the Millionth Circle, meme or whatever it is, in that I had this idea that we're really moving from being so scared and fear-based into sacred. When I heard you mention the word sacred it's moving from scared to sacred, the more of us that are really focusing on all of these conscious memes the more we create more sacredness in our culture.

Deborah: Yes and when you look at the evolution of cultures you realize that the progression of moving from the fear to actually being exposed, I was thinking of that when I first began in circles of having this big wave come over me of what a healing it is that we can now, in this day and age, come together as women in the safety and openness of being in those sacred circles where there was a healing going on. Hopefully, as a society we are progressing in many ways that we could reflect back and see that we're creating those more positive sacred movements.

When I started the circle move women's circles I didn't really know what a women's circle was. I just started meeting one amazing woman after another and I wondered what it would be like to bring all these women together under the same roof at the same time and do it in circle. It was shortly after that I started being given these books that were about women's circles, creating sacred circles and I looked to see when most of them were published. They were published in 98' when I got that nudge to start my own circles. So I realized that I was part of something much larger, like a spirituality movement that was happening organically and that is a huge part of a conscious meme is those organic movements and becoming aware that you're a part of something that's much bigger that has a positive effect.

Harmony: Sometimes things that aren't so great help start movements. I know with the Self-Care Revolution™, Robyn really held onto wow, our healthcare system is really failing. We have one out of three people getting cancer. Children are sick all over the place and wanting to change that reality has become important. I think there are more people who are jumping on the band wage saying yes, the way we do it is broken and now we need to do it in a different way.

Deborah: Yes and memeing preventative health, that has become meme.

Harmony: I was thinking while you talked about your friends Sedena and George Cappannelli and one of the things I read in their book was *Do No Go Quietly* is that 70-90% of money you will spend on healthcare in your life gets spent in the latter years of your life. I was thinking wow, self-care is so important for us to be putting time, energy and resources on the front end of our lives, so hopefully we live more peaceful existence as we go on.

Deborah: Yes.

Harmony: So lots of beautiful memeing happening with all of us.

Robyn: I love memeing.

Deborah: We have started with our Conscious Meme Network, when we are exposing something that's going on out there we're saying you've just been memed by the Conscious Meme Network. Pretty soon that will be a phrase that's memed and people won't just say what is a meme or why should we care if we've been memed?

Harmony: Are you highlighting conscious memes or unconscious memes when you meme someone?

Deborah: We're highlighting conscious memes.

Harmony: That's what I thought. You've just been memed.

Deborah: The meme awareness piece is to educate people on what a meme is and why they should care. Then the conscious meme movement is highlighting the positive organizations and movements and products and trends and ideas that are going on out there and helping to spread them even more.

Harmony: You're totally inspiring me, because inspired by the Self-Care Revolution™ over this last year, I am developing a product called soulful self-care which is all processes, activities, things that take one-two minutes that are acts of self-care that bring you back into the present moment. I thought, how fun would that be to have that be developed as a conscious meme that says take one minute right now for you and an hour later, okay take one more minute for you and have it be self-care much broader than when most people think about taking a bath or getting a massage or having a cup of tea.

Deborah: While you were talking about that I started thinking about the sound of Tibetan bells and the affect that has on people. Before I'd start a circle maybe everyone would be yakking all over and all I'd have to do is come out and gently touch those bells or maybe at an event and suddenly everyone gets quiet. There was something about what you were sharing about your own product that I thought, what if people started just having that and taking a pause.

Robyn: Deborah, can you share with everyone how they can become part of your conscious meme network?

Deborah: Thank you. We have a movement on Facebook, so all you need to do is put in Conscious Meme Movement in your Facebook search bar. We'll show up and if you click like then you'll be a part of being kept up on some of the awesome positive things that are going on out there and inspiring even phrases. Just be a part of the movement, our Conscious Meme Network is on the Internet at the website ConsciousMeme.com. We have a YouTube channel, The Conscious Meme Network, and all these links are also on our website, so that's easy.

As I mentioned earlier, we just launched the Meme Messenger E-zine and you'll want to be part of that because you'll be kept up on and connected through direct links with a lot of the positive organizations and movements and trends and products out there. We have the Self-Care Revolution™ on there and you'll be featured on every issue of that magazine, Robyn, because you are a conscious meme movement. We hope everyone will sign up.

Robyn: Thank you and it's the highlight of this interview because I love how it's grown. It's like this sweet little light of expansive energy, this consciousness...

Harmony: It feels like Deborah's energy.

Robyn: Yes.

Deborah: Thank you, and I have to say that I was so pleased at the end of last year, because Katie Couric actually memed meme to the masses by having a special on about the memes of 2012. I had to thank her for putting that word out mainstream.

I just had a beautiful Coopers Hawk fly in front of my window in the Santa Fe sky, how beautiful it was.

Robyn: Deborah, could you give us what a self-care day looks like for you, being a positive person and a person who's living a life of memeing and passion and compassion?

Deborah: I love being asked that question because I have to say that moving to Santa Fe 8 years ago from Los Angeles where I lived for 25 years, I realized how important it was for me to honor my own pace and it seems like being more immersed in nature here and having it so much more accessible, has become a huge part of my self-care. I have an area on our land that I call my circle of trees and sometimes when I'm thinking I need to do this and having to do that, I hear an inner voice nudging me to get out there and sit down in that circle of trees and take a pause.

Then I move from there in a more centered connected space and the self compassion has been a new thing for me, because I've never had a hard time being that way towards others. If I'm feeling weepy or anxious, oftentimes that's a sign for me that I'm tired and I need to take a nap. So even if I'm in my car I may pull over and lay the seat down and take 10 deep breaths. Nature is definitely one of my huge self-care pieces.

Robyn: Nature is definitely one of the core foundations of self-care.

Deborah: I also want to add, taking a look at how much joy and bliss and glee you're allowing yourself in your life, because just having that awareness of, wait am I having fun yet? Then doing something about it if that's possible, that's important self-care.

Robyn: Any final words of wisdom with our wonderful self-care revolutionaries.

Deborah: I love what we were just talking about, so that piece is the most important. I want to repeat again that quote from Richard Brody's book, that meme awareness can improve the quality of our lives and if you can carry that awareness with you and that thought as you're moving about in your lives, you can have an effect because you are it.

Robyn: That's beautiful. I'm thinking about this because we're going to end this fabulous hour with you. Deborah thank you so much for all that you've shared with us.

[End of Interview]

BILL PARRAVANO

TheKneePainGuru.com; KneesForLife.com | The Knee Pain Guru, his teachings are based on what he calls the *5 Pillars for a Pain-Free Life*.

HOW COMFORT CAN IMPROVE YOUR KNEE PAIN

[These statements have not been evaluated by the Food and Drug Administration. The information on this audiocast is not intended to diagnose, treat, cure, or prevent any disease.]

Robyn: Hello everyone and welcome to month 12 of the Self-Care Revolution™. We love this month's theme of Pay It Forward. We just listened to the lovely Deborah Koppel Mitchell to learn all about conscious memes and if you didn't get to hear it, please listen to the replay. What is a meme? It's an idea whose time has come. She talked about conscious memes that are health related, like how important it is to do burst training. She talked about Pay It Forward being a meme and many other examples.

My name is Robyn Benson and I'm a Doctor of Oriental Medicine, the Founder of Santa Fe Soul Health and Healing Center and the Host of Self-Care Revolution™. I'm feeling so much gratitude for being at the 12-month mark of this revolution, knowing that it has touched so many thousands of people's lives. Today we are interviewing Bill Parravano, who is known as The Knee Guru. Welcome for being with us today.

Bill: Hi Robyn.

Robyn: Bill has a great Pay It Forward message when it comes to knee health, which many of us know the magnificent work of Louise Hay, who talks about injuries and trauma. Pain in the knees has to do energetically with the fear of moving forward in life. As I was saying, the Self-Care Revolution™ is a movement to create awareness around the known idea that through self-care we cannot only save lives but also help prevent and reverse some illnesses from occurring in the first place. Our big message is that self-care is the true healthcare and we know that if people practice this in everyday life, from their knees to their organs, their vision and how they're feeding themselves everyday as well as how they're moving their body's, that this plays such an essential role in how you live your life and for many, how you rock your mission.

Many of us here that are Self-Care Revolutionaries, we care to take care of ourselves because we have a lot to do in this lifetime. With that I'm joined by my lovely co-host for today...

Harmony: Hi, I'm Harmony West and I'm a family health and wellness educator, here at Santa Fe Soul Health and Healing Center. I'm very excited to be involved in interviewing Bill.

Robyn: Bill, I'm so glad I've had time to speak with you prior to our call today. Bill, The Knee Pain Guru, will give you the life-long solution to the pain in your knees. Say No to Knee Replacement is the distillation of his life's work over the past 14 years. It is a cutting-edge template that is key to eliminating chronic knee pain. Using a holistic approach, Bill's teachings are based on what he calls the 5 Pillars for a Pain-Free Life:

- Water,

- Breathing,

- Nutrition,

- Sleep, and

- Stretching

Bill has traveled worldwide, bringing comfort and relief to thousands of people.

I know there is so much more to learn about you, so I just want to add that as an instructor Bill has taught 30 osteopathic physicians in the Ukraine and has had such success that he is now offering his knowledge to a much larger audience. He is here and ready to share his knowledge and experience. This information can shorten the healing process and improve your quality of life. There is hope and change can happen. He has seen the healing effects time and time again and is more equipped than ever to help you find the results you so desperately need. In his own words, Bill describes his goal to get the world a natural option for surgery, where everyone is comfortable in their body and can enjoy strong healthy joints that last a lifetime.

That sounds good to me. Welcome Bill, again I'm so glad to have you with us and I must say I've been a practicing Doctor of Oriental Medicine for 21 years and have treated thousands of knees. I do injections to help restore knee integrity in a natural way to bring back the nature of the knee.

Harmony: Bill, how big of a problem is knee pain? Do lots of people have problems with their knees?

Bill: Yes. Just to give you an idea. On the website of American Academy of Orthopedic Surgeons in 2011, there were 676,000 knee replacement surgeries done in the U.S. alone. That's staggering, and of course that number is exponentially bigger worldwide and that's just the people whose knees have degenerated to a point where they feel like they have no other options. So you can imagine how a person that's looking at a knee replacement at the age of 60-80 years old has already been suffering for 20-30 years with knee pain and felt like they had no other options.

We're looking at a huge amount of people that experience knee pain and whenever I have a conversation with someone about what I do, that I train people's bodies to eliminate chronic knee pain, they either say they have knee pain or someone they know has it.

Harmony: Why are so many people in pain? Why does there seem to be an epidemic of knee pain?

Bill: I think it's a combination of an outmoded way of looking at the body and not knowing what the new mode is. What is the new way of looking at the body? I look at everything from a nervous system level. It's the hardwiring we have which connects the physical with the non-physical and that nervous system is entrained in a way that's designed to protect us and keep us safe. It also protects us from changing, so when we introduce something different to the nervous system, it wants to go back to what it already knows. Think about it, why change is so difficult. Anything in our lives that we want to change we have to setup habits around that to support us, to support that change for taking place.

Harmony: So do people have really bad habits to begin with?

Bill: I don't necessarily know that it's bad habits I just think that sometimes it's just tweaks that need to be made. Like sometimes I've had clients that I've worked with that say their knees hurt. I ask them how much water they drink and they're like, does coffee count? Does soda count? Does tea count? I'm like no I'm talking about plain water. Well, I don't know I don't really drink that much water. Well let's try this week; you start drinking half your body weight in ounces of water per day and let's see how that changes. I've had clients come back to me and say "that worked" and their knee pain went away as a result of just drinking water.

Robyn: Can you give us a background on how you even got into this?

Bill: Fast. In 1998, I dislocated my left knee the first of four times, skiing. I had gone with a friend skiing and was going down the first hill and there was powder snow and ice together and I did one of those snowplow things. I hadn't skied much in my life and was doing that where the tips of my skis were together and the ski that was downhill slid out and the ski that was uphill stuck and I face planted, and in the process my knee popped and I tore the ligament in my left knee.

Harmony: So you got to experience what the medical establishment knows how to do to fix that knee?

Bill: Right. I really want to be clear in my message, that I'm supportive of the existing medical model when it's appropriate. If I'm in a car accident or if I decide to face plant with skis on my feet and tear the ligament in my knees then I want them in my corner. I want them to fix what's broken or torn, but when there's nothing broken or torn and we're just looking at pain, at the experience in the nervous system, then I don't believe the conventional medical model has any idea of how to really address the person and bring them back to being whole again.

Robyn: Continue on with your journey and your initial injury and how you've been doing this, how it's taken you around the world and maybe give us an example of how you do your training with people. What are the pillars you speak of that are the foundation of your teaching.

Bill: I not only dislocated my knee that time skiing but I dislocated it three more times in judo, volleyball and softball, before I pulled my head out of the sand and said I probably should go to the doctor and get this checked out. When I went to the doctor, a great orthopedic surgeon for the University of Louisville sports teams, Dr. John Ellis. He looked at my knee and said you tore your ACL, what would you like to do? He said you're 29 years old, so you're at the age where you can go either way. If I wanted to lead a sedative lifestyle the rest of my life it would have been you don't need your ACL you can completely function or if you're going to be athletic and you want to do a lot of things, than get the operation.

I went a month later, had the operation where they did a patella replacement, which is where they take part of my patella tendon and recreate the ligament in my knee. The surgery went great. They took out two pieces of meniscus as well. I did three months of physical therapy and I was at the end of what the medical model was able to help me with. The knee was mechanically sound. The left leg was as strong as the right, but I still had swelling, pain and tension in my left knee as well as in the rest of my body as a result of compensating for my knee and that set me on the path I'm on right now.

I ended up selling a computer company that I owned in Louisville, Kentucky at the time and in that I traveled for two and a half years studying all the things that I wanted to do to bring my body back into balance. I got involved in bodywork. I got involved in nutrition. I read as many books as I could. That was like pulling the pieces together to help me, like what was the next step to help myself, and my body to feel normal again? In that period of time I rode a bicycle across the country from Seattle to the Kentucky/West Virginia border. I spent five months traveling around Europe studying martial arts and bodywork. I saw different perspectives from different cultures and understanding what it really takes to get the body to a place where the knee felt like part of my body again.

It was 2002 when I stopped traveling and began working on clients in the Louisville, Kentucky area as a way of sharing the knowledge and information that I had, which I'd gained from traveling for 2 ½ years, and finding a lot of real world experience. Okay this stuff works on me, so how does it work on someone else that's not me and see the kinds of results that I would get.

Harmony: Did you already know at that time Bill, that you wanted to help other people or were you still exclusively on your own healing journey?

Bill: That's a great question. I was definitely on my own healing journey in realizing that my healing journey was starting to include other people.

Robyn: You were paying it forward right? This is a beautiful story.

Bill: It's like my big love was judo. I just wanted to get my knee back so I could go compete in judo again. I love throwing people. I'd get up in the morning and that's all I could think about. So my healing was about getting back and getting on the judo mat again so I could throw people.

Harmony: That's so cute.

Bill: There is never a loss of injured bodies in a judo dojo. I was seeing people who had something going on with their shoulders, their knee, their hips or something like that and after practice I'd say hey Brad, come over here and let me take a look at that. Let me look at that toe, the ankle, knee or the hip. I started working with these things and I found that I was getting some amazing results in a short period of time. I was still on my journey to give back, so I can do judo again, but at the same time it was expanding out like this is a really cool trick, let me show you. That's how it started to grow.

Robyn: Did you get a degree with all this learning you did? I'm curious.

Bill: I was certified by the Society of Ortho-Bionomy International, which is a style of bodywork. I got certified in both the U.S. and Europe.

Robyn: Cool.

Harmony: So, did you start putting together the ideas that you were learning during your traveling? Did you start compiling them into some type of cohesive form? Tell us about developing the five pillars for a pain-free life. Those sound wonderful.

Bill: I learned a style of bodywork, which is absolutely phenomenal, I think the world of it, but I also saw its limitations. It was like okay, taking the body to a position of comfort, which is the principles of Ortho-Bionomy was an amazing approach to getting the body to heal itself, but there were limitations to that and we needed to look at a broader perspective. The body is supposed to be made up of 80% water, so how does water play a role? When you put the body in comfort how does that play a role in the body healing? Looking at that and nutrition, because as I mentioned before I'm looking at everything from a nervous system level.

How does the electrical system in the bodywork? If we don't have good conductivity of the electrical impulses coming from the brain to the rest of the body then the body isn't going to be able to heal. So what are those factors that go into it? We look at...

- Water,

- Breathing,

- Nutrition,

- Sleep, and

- Stretching

We look into all these elements to see how they're used in order for the body to heal itself and realize that if we leave out different aspects of these components that the body uses to heal, we leave a lot on the table. So, I'm using myself as a guinea pig. I use my judo buddies and I'm starting to see clients and say how did this change when you start adding these other elements in? We started getting some pretty miraculous results.

Robyn: I think this is great. Being a doctor of Chinese medicine, this is like the foundation of how I like to look at the body. We are electrical beings, before our biology and chemistry even works. In fact, Harmony and I were both speakers in month 5, which has to do with earthing, electro-sanitizing your life and growing your own garden. Just to talk about how critical it is that we're in this healthy electrical field at all times. I think it's great that the work you're doing is educating people as you said earlier, in much of what our medical system leaves out and getting back to the fundamentals of nature and how our bodies are like the earth in many ways.

In this whole path of studying, going to Europe and learning about Ortho-Bionomy and all of that, what was so revolutionary outside of these 5 pillars? What was your ultimate aha? Now that you know what you know, would you have chosen not to do the ACL surgery repair?

Bill: Yes. That's a good question. No one has ever asked me that before. My big aha was while I attended a workshop in Chicago presented by Ortho-Bionomy. Whenever any instructor was teaching anything remotely close to the knee, I was the person on the table and I remember they were doing what's called an external femur rotation, which is the bone in the upper leg being rotated externally, which is to the outside of the body. I got on the table, the instructor did a simple move taking the bone in my upper leg out a little more and held it there for a minute or two and then let my leg go and asked me to get up and share with the group what happened.

I remember getting up and standing and was in completely disbelief as I looked down at the scar on my knee which when they do a patella replacement is dead center on the knee joint, so it's virtually impossible to kneel down without kneeling on the scar tissue and it's extremely painful. When I looked down at the scar it had shifted a ¼ inch in the matter of a couple minutes. There was this utter wave of relief that came over me and I remember breaking down in tears because I could actually bend and kneel down now, because the scar had shifted enough and that really solidified in my brain that my path needed to be different from what I had been doing.

Robyn: What did you do that shifted the scar?

Bill: When the surgery was done the scar is dead center on the knee cap but my body was holding onto a tension pattern in the bone that caused the entire leg to be shifted in a way that when that tension was released, caused the entire pattern in my leg to change and as a result the scar shifted. The way I knelt before this release took place in my femur was completely different.

Robyn: So rather than focusing on the healing of the knee you looked at the connection to the femur in terms of healing.

Bill: The other question you asked is would I have had the surgery again? I have a friend, Sean Stevenson, who put together a program for me called Regrow Your Knees. It's a nutritional protocol made up of Chinese herbs, medicinal mushrooms and super foods that have the ability to recreate neural pathways in the body and regrow cartilage, meniscus, tendons and ligaments. When you posed that question as to whether I would have the surgery again knowing what I know now, that's a toss up.

There are parts of me that look and I go gosh I wonder what that would have been like if I'd have gone on a nutritional protocol to see how that could have changed what was going on in my knee. So there's a question in my mind; however, at the same time I do not regret having the surgery because it allowed me to have access to my life again. The fear I had about taking a step and my knee popping out of joint and me lying on the ground clutching my knee screaming because it popped out of joint, it's an awful feeling. I wouldn't wish it on anyone and just to have that confidence in my mind to know that my knee joint is mechanically sound and the ligaments are in tact and the limitation isn't in my body anymore it's in my mind.

Robyn: I'm so fascinated being a practicing Doctor of Oriental Medicine where my special really is sports medicine. The idea that you say come see me, because a lot of people once they get to the point where they need a knee replacement there really is no other choice. I certainly have my thoughts on that, but that's an audacious statement and I'd love to see how you answer that. If someone calls you as a result of this call, how do you address it? Can you go into more detail of how you can prevent a knee replacement? This is the path you've taken which has been effective, so go for it.

Bill: The piece with bone on bone is that the structure of the body has been compromised. The body is a tensegrity structure. Buckminster Fuller made it famous, like Epcot center or a geodesic dome, where the structure is created by the tension within the structure and if the structure is compromised it means the tension has shifted to another part of the structure. Consequently, when a person has a bone on bone situation they have extremely tight hips and a lower back and what happens as a result of the tension, frequently from sitting a lot, the tension is then thrown into the knees, so the knee joint must compensate for the lack of flexibility in the hips and lower back.

That compromises the tensegrity structure and as a result, the joint then begins to wear because every time they take a step there's no shock-absorption taking place in the body. So as we begin to reestablish the tensegrity structure by loosening up the hips and lower back, getting the tension pattern and relieving the pain in the knee joint, now the body begins to elongate and it gets more in line with gravity. So every time you're taking a step, the shock that was going to the knees is now distributed evenly throughout the rest of the structure.

When you look at the body globally like that you begin to understand that the bone on bone situation can be reversed, I believe, by setting up those conditions that allow the body to heal itself. Start by creating comfort and simultaneously while you're creating comfort you look at water, nutrition, inflammation in the body, breathing and mindset. All those things create the conditions so the body is able to move from a place of being in pain and degenerating to a place of being comfortable and regenerating itself.

Robyn: That's great, so the main thing that you're doing with your patients in terms of hands on is this Ortho-Bionomy, right?

Bill: I'm teaching them to do this for themselves over the Internet.

Robyn: Wow!

Bill: That's what's really cool about it.

Robyn: That's awesome. So through doing a Skype session?

Bill: Yes, I do Skype sessions with clients. We work one-on-one, where we get on a call and they basically outline what happened to them, where their knees hurt, when they hurt and what they're doing in their lives. Then we systematically begin to create the conditions in their life and body that are preventing their bodies from healing itself. The body defaults to healing it knows how to heal, so we don't have to ask it to do so. We don't have to ask it to pump blood. We don't have to ask it to process oxygen or breathe while you sleep, because it knows how to do that. Healing is the same way so if the body isn't healing the person is doing something to prevent their body from healing itself.

So we start removing those blocks that's preventing the body from healing and adding in the things that allows the body to heal itself and the magic happens. The body does it on its own.

Harmony: When you talk about bringing the body back to a place of comfort, can you talk a bit more about that? Are you talking about its natural healthful state?

Bill: Good question. I was just asked about this just an hour ago. Comfort is always changing and there is optimal comfort, like if you wake up from a really good nights sleep and your body feels light and loose and free, that's ultimate comfort. There's also comfort within the discomfort and when a knee is in pain, let's say it's 80%, so the knee has 8 out of 10 the pain is in the knee. If we can create enough comfort in the knee joint to tell the nervous system to let go of the tension pattern that's going on in the knee to bring the pain level down to a seven or six, then we've succeeded. Because, what we're doing even though the pain is not completely gone from the joint, we're re-educating the nervous system how to heal on its own.

We're taking the body from a sympathetic nervous system state, a fight or flight state, and getting it into a parasympathetic state or a rest and relax state, which is where the body heals. Even though we've only moved from an 8 to a 7 or a 6, relatively speaking we've created comfort in the joint and we've begun to move the body to a place where it has more leverage to heal itself, like we're getting a foot in the door so to speak. As we create more comfort in the body, and going from an 8 to a 7 or 6 today, let's revisit this tomorrow. So now the pain may have gone to a 7. We create comfort again and we bring it down to a 5 and we do that every day, day in day out, teaching the body how to understand what comfort is and the body then does it on its own.

It can sleep better. Make sure the water and nutrition is there. Make sure you're breathing properly. All those factors go into easily moving the body to a place of healing itself and being out of pain.

Harmony: So you're taking your knowledge of Ortho-Bionomy and customizing stretches and ways that the body can go back to its natural state of comfort, as well as adding in nutrition, water and the other pillars is that correct?

Bill: That's correct.

Harmony: Can you talk about breathing a bit? I mean, everybody breathes but it sounds like you mean something really different.

Bill: I've been involved in a martial art called Sistema; it's a Russian martial art. One of my instructors is Mikhail Raipcal. He's in the Russian military and he was asked at a seminar how important breathing was. He calmly looked at the person and said well, if you don't breathe you die. That really sums up the importance of breathing, right there.

Harmony: But you must do something that's a bit more specific than that or do you just tell people to deep breathe.

Bill: The body when it's in pain wants to default to holding its breath and making the breath short. In Sistema there is an approach to breathing and breathing is defined in Sistema as a smooth flow of air in through the nose and out through the mouth. The more you breathe the more you relax the nervous system. The more you bring the body from that fight or flight state to the rest and relax state and many times people with knee pain, when they're getting up out of a chair will hold their breath, begin to get out of the chair and when they've fully stood up then they start breathing again.

What ends up happening is that creates a pattern in the nervous system to expect the pain whenever they move. Sistema sandwiches the movement between the breath so you initiate the movement with the breath and you finish the movement with the breath. So if you begin to even think to get up out of a chair you start breathing in through your nose and out your mouth. So the movement is initiated with the breath. You begin to stand up continuing to breathe, smooth flow of air and then after you've fully stood up you're continuing to breathe. So now you've relaxed the tension in your nervous system, you've relaxed your body as you're getting up out of the chair. You can extrapolate that out to any movement you do.

Getting in and out of bed.

Getting up and down from the floor.

Reaching into the washer and dryer.

Picking up your children.

The breathing is all-applicable in any situation. Bringing that awareness and understanding of when we hold our breath is so enlightening in terms of how the knees can begin to feel different when we incorporate that simple concept of breath to movement.

Harmony: It seems like it's a natural human design or something that when you're in pain to contract and hold your breath and try to get small, but what you're doing is bringing awareness almost to the antithesis of that, to breathe and bring your awareness right here instead of running away from the pain.

Bill: Right. You got it.

Harmony: Would you switch a little now to talk about nutrition? What are some of the nutritional ideas that you give people to support them with their knees?

Bill: I'm very much along the lines of what you both teach. I believe the more we can get to natural… ideally if we could forage it or grow it ourselves that that would be ideal and best, but when that's not possible then I'd be looking at farmer's markets. Know the person that's growing your food.

Harmony: So whole vegetables, whole foods and whole fruits?

Bill: Yes. I'm along the lines thinking of Paleo, less than price, somewhere around in there.

Robyn: I'm with you 100%. I just want to say too that I love in your work and that you're sharing with your clients that it's self-care. You're teaching them through the Internet ultimately and yet they have to do it and that's a big message. We seem to want to delegate a lot of our life to others, pills, pharmaceuticals and that's such a foundational message of the Self-Care Revolution™ is returning to nature, because it can solve a lot of our issues.

Harmony: What I'm making out that much of the work that you do with people has deeper more, far reaching affect than just their knees.

Bill: Very much so.

Harmony: So whole foods, anything else nutrition-wise? Do you get into omegas, fish oils or super foods? So are you trying to get people away from boxed processed foods and into whole foods?

Bill: That question is all over the board depending on the person I'm working with and where they are in their journey. To be honest I work with some clients that I don't even touch the nutrition piece. Sometimes it's really crazy because their belief system, be it... food is so tied to religion and nationality and culture and so many other things that are so deeply ingrained that to start talking about how someone needs to eat this or not eat that can get touchy. I see where clients are and support them where they are. I've gotten people out of knee pain without ever changing a thing in their diets. That is not ideally how I would like things to go but everybody...

Harmony: You're meeting people where they are.

Bill: Right. I do use some supplementation. I do look at fish oil and magnesium supplements because I think that's beneficial. I look at some homeopathic remedies as a way of dealing with swelling and inflammation locally within the knee. I think the big piece, no matter where it comes from, whether nutrition or supplementation or different things people can do to eliminate the inflammation in the body, which seems to be the big crutch people have in terms of not only their knees but also their life. So whatever we can begin doing to eliminate the gut inflammation, gives the body an incredible amount of leverage in healing itself.

Robyn: Can you talk to the people who don't understand inflammation, what it is and why the gut might play a part in that?

Bill: When I talk about knee pain and inflammation, most people think my knee isn't swollen or the problem is just in my knee, so they're looking too close to the issue and not looking systemically at what is going on in the entire body that's contributing to the knee. The way I look at it the knee is just the weakest link in a series of tension from the head to the feet. When the knee is injured or hurt, like when I tore the ligament in my knee, there was already tension patterns pulling in the rest of my body way too tight that manifested in the knee and created the knee.

So I believe in looking systemically and food and gut inflammation is looking systemically as how we absorb the nutrition that we get from our food and if we aren't capable of absorbing the nutrition it's difficult for the body to send that nutrition to the knee and heal it.

Robyn: That's a big part of Chinese medicine too is the health of the gut. It's where we produce our neurotransmitters in terms of our feel good hormones. It's true that leaky gut syndrome that's so prevalent with our SAD (standard American diet), causes major micro molecules to get out of the intestinal walls and into the body and cause a lot of inflammation and then we just keep feeding it. I think it's fantastic. How successful have you been? I mean, with your clientele and preventing them from having knee replacement?

Bill: I've had a lot of success, but that success was dependent on the mindset of the person I'm working with. A lot of times clients will come and they're like well, I'll try it out for a few weeks or a month and I'm like no, that won't work. We have to fully commit and look at all the fears, doubts and concerns first and get them addressed and off the table before we can start moving forward. When I get a client that is willing to fully step across that line and commit to their own well-being, then I have phenomenal results.

Many times a diagnosis of bone on bone and someone needing a knee replacement, the doctors honestly don't know what else to say. They only have so many categories that they can fit people in, to help them get out of pain. It's prescription drugs, painkilling shots or a knee replacement surgery if it's far enough down the road. When a client has heard that, it's almost like a death sentence, where you're going to need a knee replacement. They become that diagnosis and buy into it so heavily that any other option isn't really feasible.

So, what I like to do once we get all the conditions setup and the client begins to see results, the results become addictive. It's like oh wow, my knee feels this good after only a week. It feels this good after three weeks. How good can this get? By just focusing on comfort and creating the conditions so the body can heal itself, the body easily and effortlessly moves to a place of recovery or regeneration.

Harmony: Can you talk about sleep for a few minutes? I notice that's one of your five pillars and I think we're a sleep deprived nation. Would you be willing to talk about that and how you support people?

Bill: Absolutely. That's where we recover is when we sleep. When the body is experiencing chronic pain it's continually looking for the threat. So what happens is when it's looking for the threat, one of the things the body isn't capable of is getting sufficient sleep, because it's in a fight or flight mode. Therefore, the more comfort we can get the body into the more of a rest and relax, parasympathetic state we can get the body into the better capable the body is of sleeping, resting and recovering and it all happens when we sleep.

Harmony: So sleep is super important for us to be able to recover and rest. Do people fight you with that or do most say okay, I get it I need to sleep more?

Bill: Different people are in different places. Most people like sleeping. However, most people with knee pain either have difficulty sleeping or they're so Type-A personality driven that it's difficult for them to get to sleep or stay asleep. They get into a dog chasing their tail mode. I want to get out of pain so I work harder to try to get out of pain but working harder gets me into more pain so I can't get out of pain so I have to work harder. They get into this vicious cycle that creates the conditions for them to have a knee replacement surgery when they're old enough.

If we interrupt that cycle and create comfort in that cycle, and teach the body how to rest and relax and recover, then instead of it being an upward spiral of pain, swelling, inflammation, etc. we go down that spiral and we begin to create comfort, more relaxation, more awareness, etc.

Robyn: That's such a great word, comfort, and I love how that's a big part of your message here. How long do these steps take that you're teaching people, in terms of eliminating their knee pain and these secrets to strong healthy knee joints that you're sharing with your clientele? What are you looking at, people spending 10-15 minutes a day doing that?

Bill: Clients I'd say spend 10-15 minutes in the morning and again in the evening working on these concepts and principles and they can see tremendous results. I was speaking with a client earlier today, Edward, that I've been working with for a month and a half and he was saying Bill, I was sitting in church with my family and my knee was bothering me. He said I just reached down and did that little thing you showed me in your video and I didn't have to get up or do anything, it was right there while I was sitting down in church. I said that's perfect. That's what I'm talking about it doesn't have to be like a separate part of your life. I want these to be tools in your toolbox that you pull out when you need them and where you need them so you can go on and live your life, because pain is going to happen your entire life.

It's a function of stress and tension that builds up in the body and the ability to diffuse that stress and tension in the body. So the more we could train our nervous system how to kick off that stress and tension faster, the better results we're going to get, the better recovery time we're going to get.

Robyn: I love the acronym you have for pain (pay attention to internal nurturing). I think that's much of what you're sharing with learning how to walk and have proper posture, which is a big part of how energy is moving in our electrical system. I think it's fantastic what you're sharing.

Harmony: Everything he's doing is self-care.

Robyn: That's right, rather than people getting this diagnosis and overreacting instead of being proactive and seeing the knee guru and very often choose surgery. I see a lot of people who are not happy. Like what happened to you, even though you had your ACL repair it took months to recover and my husband two years ago had the same thing and he had a major surgery. He's a big time skier and I was trying to encourage him not to do the surgery and he is like, I have to have surgery because I want to get back on the slopes, that means more to me than anything.

It's interesting because for two months he didn't have the surgery because he had to get the inflammation down so we worked on that, but ultimately its his choice and it's amazing two years later the amount of rehab that he still does like hot yoga twice a week because he's so stiff with scar tissue and all that. I like how you talk about all the mindset and this is a big question regarding that. If people really want to go the natural route and be patient and do this relearning that you did for 2 ½ years, reeducating yourself, not knowing even half that stuff before starting on your journey.

I also think about the fact that you've had your surgery and you're still on this quest. It's very interesting that in the end right now you say that you're glad you had the surgery, but regardless of that, that it put you on this path to be a messenger to let people know you're paying it forward by sharing all the information you've learned to ultimately say that so many people can reverse their knee pain, which is a great thing because like you said it is an epidemic.

Right now can you talk about your call offer and where they can go… KneesForLife.com and sign up for a free chapter from your book?

Bill: Yes that's correct. They can go to the website and I have an offer where they can get a free chapter from my book and an audio of the three biggest mistakes knee pain sufferers make and how to avoid them.

Robyn: Can you tell us what those three mistakes are?

Bill: It has to hurt to heal. You have to work hard to get the knee out of pain. It's going to take a long time for the knee to heal.

Harmony: And none of those are really true?

Bill: No.

Robyn: If someone had an ACL injury right now, based on your knowledge and all the rehab you've helped your patients receive through their own self-care, today would you recommend surgery? Do you feel like people can avoid arthroscopic surgeries that are going on?

Bill: Arthroscopic, sure. If something is broken or torn it's going to be a case by case basis, because is the ligament partially or fully torn? Is the meniscus a big tear or a small one? I think a good 80-90% of surgeries that take place today could be avoided. They don't need to happen. I was on a call earlier today with a client who worked with my program for four months and she got great results but she was limited to how she was able to extend her leg by the chunk of meniscus that's torn in her knee. So, I spoke to her and said Suzie, if I were you I'd just go do it. It would be an outpatient procedure that you'll have done and in a month you can continue the principles o f my program and you'll be good to go. You can do it nutritionally and avoid the surgery, but I have no idea how long it will take.

Harmony: It sounds like you're very realistic with your clients too. That's wonderful.

Robyn: Can you also talk about your upgrade bonus for our listeners? This is very generous.

Bill: Sure. I'm offering, for anyone who would like to sign up for my program, that I will spend an hour with them, going over their individual situation with their knees and giving them a step-by-step strategy of what I would do within my program to get them out of the pain the quickest for whatever their situation is. I'll custom tailor the program so they can get out of pain the fastest.

Robyn: What's the best way for people to get in touch with you?

Bill: That would be to shoot me an email at Bill@thekneepainguru.com.

Robyn: You've created a lot of content for your clients and offers. You have products for people, is there one final comment… let's say for 100 people who might listen to this in the next few days that have knee pain, what's one nugget that you've learned in the last 10 years that you'd like to share.

Bill: I think the big thing is that there's always a solution. I look at the body and it's like it doesn't have to be like that there's another solution. I want to share that. It gives people hope that there are options out there and the fear we go into limits the number of options, so if you take a moment and see things without the fear you'll see all the options and opportunities that will open up.

Robyn: That's a good ending note. There is always a solution. Today where there's so much stress and people are feeling so depressed and anxious and overwhelmed, to know there's always a solution.

Harmony: They need to come to Bill and he has 101.

Robyn: Thank you for the work you're doing in the world and to really help people solve this pain in the knee issue. That's your story so we support you in your self-care message in helping people take charge of their lives because like any of us know, for me as a Doctor of Oriental Medicine and Harmony and the work she does with her clients, ultimately we're just facilitators and this is the big message of self-care… it's time to take care of yourself like never before. Thank you.

[End of Interview]

CHARLEY JOHNSON

PifExperience.org | Head of the Global Pay It Forward Movement and President of the Pay It Forward Foundation

PAY IT FORWARD: THE MOVEMENT FOR ALL SEVEN-BILLION PEOPLE

[These statements have not been evaluated by the Food and Drug Administration. The information on this audiocast is not intended to diagnose, treat, cure, or prevent any disease.]

Robyn: Hello everyone and welcome to month twelve of the Self-Care Revolution™, celebrating life and paying it forward. It's been a fabulous month so far and I have to say as I listen to our theme song, that's my true Christmas carol that's in my head all the time. I think many of you that have been with us since the beginning of the year, you have memorized that first 30 seconds and we're grateful again to Chris Miller and Harold Payne, who spent several months getting that right. The message is so powerful, especially in this theme of Pay It Forward, this self-care piece of it is critical in terms of how we feel in everyday life is such a big root of how we can give our best selves to each other and the world at large.

I'm Robyn Benson, a Doctor of Oriental Medicine and Founder of Santa Fe Soul Health and Healing Center. The way I like to Pay It Forward is, 21 years of experience in working with patients one-on-one; it's such a joy to be able to give my years of experience to people and to help get people out of pain, to find their passion and to help people know what it's like to have excellent health. I'm here with…

Kevin: Hi, I'm Kevin Snow, Intuitive Counselor here at Santa Fe Soul. Definitely one of the ways that I love to Pay It Forward is by helping people create clarity where there is none. One of the things we'll talk about today with our amazing speaker is simplicity and I definitely think that makes a complex world a little simpler and one of the ways to do that is to Pay It Forward.

Robyn: On this beautiful Christmas Eve day I want to take a moment to express once again, our gratitude to all of our speakers, who in their own way have certainly suggested a Self-Care Revolution™ but they are paying forward their best information. We say they haven't held anything back and have given you what they consider to be the golden nuggets of what they need to share to help you live your best life, including our speaker today, Charley Johnson. Welcome to the Self-Care Revolution™ and thank you for being here on this special day.

Charley: Thank you for having me.

Robyn: Charley is now Head of the Global Pay It Forward Movement and President of the Pay It Forward Foundation. He's the creator of the Pay It Forward Bracelet, a physical reminder to do good that has been sent to over 2.4 million people in 132. The Official website of the Pay It Forward Movement along with the Pay It Forward Hall of Fame in November of 2011 with the First inductee being Catherine Ryan Hyde, author of the *Pay It Forward*, the Novel. Again welcome, we're so thrilled to have you with us.

Charley: Beautiful, thank you for having me.

Robyn: Charley, maybe you could explain to our audience, we have a lot of people here with us live right now, how you started this movement and maybe give us your background and how you got to this place.

Charley: I was not the beginner or starter of the movement, the phrase has been around for thousands of years. What most of the listeners and most of the audience know *Pay It Forward* from is the book and the movie; book 1999 and movie 2000 – with Kevin Spacey, Helen Hunt and Haley Joel Osment. It's got a cult following. There are lots of people that know about that phrase, what Pay It Forward is and how to become a part of it because of that book and that movie. That's how I watched it and found out about it and that's how I learned about these three little words.

I was 20 years old at the time and it struck me. I loved that you could do something for someone and just move on with life. You didn't have to wait for that awkward time when they were going to figure out how to pay you back and if they told you two weeks and it went to three the tension it caused for people when you did something for them and they had to pay you back. I loved that you could do something and just ask them to do it for someone else in the future whenever they wanted. That's what really got me stuck and clicked with me.

Robyn: How did that manifest in your life?

Charley: Around 2001 is when everything progressed into that. We didn't do anything big after that. We did what most people did we enjoyed the movie, it became part of our life, we started tipping bigger and going out of our way and we now had a phrase that we could throw towards someone and say you're grateful that I did this for you, Pay It Forward and do it for someone else. Or, you bought my coffee, you'll never see me again so do it for someone in the future when they forget their wallet and that phrase put a lot of people's minds at ease because it was easy to do something for someone and move on.

Robyn: Beautiful.

Kevin: I think the message itself since the movie, there are thousands of offshoots of this and people that have started things and possibly going different directions, so maybe you could speak a little to how that is affecting this particular movement in general and what you're doing to move it forward.

Charley: I think everything in life is about living and learning. You need to do what you feel is right at the time. After the movie and the book came out, Katherine and people promoted the book, talked about the movie and got people talking about it more and more. Like you said, hundreds if not thousands of different groups popped up and they would do their own thing, have their own website and do a Pay It Forward campaign in the school, their city, church or wherever.

Then there was the invention of social media, Facebook and Twitter and it just exploded. Now, the common man such as myself looked at that and said this is great. Everyone is talking about it. Everyone knows this phrase. There are millions across the world talking about it in hundreds of countries, so this can only be a good thing. As time goes on you start looking at very successful companies and organizations and movements and there's usually a central theme. There's usually one group that guides and as I started digging in to commit to this 100% back in 2011, I loved that people were doing things.

I never want to stop anybody from doing what they think is going to make the world better, but Coca Cola has Coca Cola, Apple has Apple, these large successful organizations have one name, one voice, one purpose and are moving in one direction. So, you have 1000 different people with 1000 different ideas heading off in 1000 different directions with 1000 different logos and 1000 different ways of what they think Pay It Forward is. So, when people find out about the book and the movie or when they see the movie and read the book or maybe they read an article about the big thing with the drive-troughs nowadays where someone buys a coffee and gives it to the person behind them.

They do a Google search and all these groups pop up. It's going all these different directions, different opinions, egos and people, and when we want people to do something good for the world or we're trying to get them excited about wanting to make today better than yesterday, if they have too many options, unfortunately they don't do anything. It kind of neutralizes and freezes them.

Robyn: Right.

Charley: Then they start wondering what to do, so I'm not going to do anything. What we've done in the past year to 18 months is we've trademarked a logo and we're trying to become that central focus, that one voice. So, when people come from all over the world and say what can I do? What is Pay It Forward? How can I get involved? How can I bring it to my city? We can give them that one direction and I believe that's helped us with our momentum.

Kevin: Awesome. We have the bracelets at our center, how would someone go about getting a bunch of those bracelets?

Charley: They can jump on our website at PifExperience.org. There's a tab on there with bracelets, which gives you information on who to email. It's a simple process to order them and we can ship all over the world.

Robyn: I love my bracelet and have been wearing it ever since we received them two weeks ago. We have them up front and in fact we're paying it forward and we're just giving them away to anyone who wants one.

Charley: The bracelet was created in 2006/2007 when Facebook was really starting to come about. I started noticing so many people buried in their phones, computers and emails, what have you so I wanted to create some physical something, something very simple that could fit around the wrist to be the reminder that it's your turn to do something good, but then also be passed on because that's the whole point of Pay It Forward. Pass that bracelet on once you do something good, so it acts as a reminder to that person and brings back that human connection, that one human being physically touching another human being and saying this is why I did this, it's your turn in the future.

Robyn: I love the logo as well, that definitely gets the message across that this is helping each other. How did you get it into all these different countries? Can you share how this all happened and where the birthing of this was in 2011?

Charley: The bracelet was back in 2007 and that's what got us into a lot of these countries. We started with a simple order of 1000 bracelets with an individual wrapper that talks about how the bracelet is used. A couple weeks later we handed them out through Utah, but we started receiving emails from Colorado, Idaho, Missouri and Texas and we noticed that people were doing what we were asking. We were seeing that the bracelets were being passed on to friends and family and strangers as they committed a random act.

So we purchased 10k, 100k, 200k, and around the 100-200k point you have enough where people would get one from Utah or Texas or somewhere here in the states and they would travel to Europe or South America, China or Asia or somewhere and then we began getting emails from different countries. We had a very simple remedial blog that talked about some stories. We didn't have any way to advertise or market. We didn't spend any money other than on the bracelets. It was all word of mouth and we started getting requests from countries we'd never heard of, so we kept buying 100k and now we're at 2.4 to 130 + countries.

Robyn: That's incredible.

Kevin: That's a great example of this concept and I think that is what is spreading this word is being the Pay It Forward message yourself. Do you have any favorite stories about emails or messages you've received?

Charley: One of my favorites that we always talk about is probably in late 2011. Once the new website was up and people started noticing there was an organization and we were kicking in 100% of our time to this, a lady wanted to share her story and get it on the website to let the world see it. A random day walking through on her way to work, a construction worker walked up to her and handed her a flower and said I just wanted to make your day better. He didn't hit on her. He wasn't trying to sell her anything. He wasn't doing anything out of the blue that a typical guy would do to a woman.

He simply felt an urge to make someone smile. As you sat there and listened to this lady talk about her story, you could hear the emotion in her voice. She had to take a break and you could sense there was emotion and probably tears on the other end. It was a random day but she could tell us everything about that day. She could tell us the time of day, the temperature, what she was wearing, how her hair was made up and how she was feeling.

What we like to do with these stories is give them a frame or time of reference and I was thinking that the way she was telling the story this was somewhat of a just happened type of story, but it happened like 30 years earlier. That is when things clicked for me, that if you ask a human being, if I asked you to when you bought your house, when you got that new car or an amount of money you thought was going to make you happy, most likely you won't be able to tell me within a week, a month or even a year of when that happened.

But, we all have that day when some random guy/girl came out of the blue for no other reason except to help you. You were having a bad day and someone made it better and we remember that. That's something that's burned into our brain. When that lady told us her story it's always something we talk about in interviews and is something we share because of how long ago it happened and how much emotion still popped up in her voice talking about it.

Kevin: I can feel it even as you're telling the story. I can feel that level of emotion. It taps into those instances in my own life as well.

Charley: Yes.

Kevin: I'm wondering what's happening right now with the movement.

Charley: What's happening now… just a lot of emails and questions, interviews and spreading the word. There's a lot of working with the people who have come to us in the last few years to get the movement into their city or country and helping them with questions as well as getting more people involved. There is quite the momentum going on with larger news organizations talking about it. The New York Times, MSNBC, larger organizations are doing articles or are speaking about Pay It Forward. However, the problem is and I'd like to bring these up so we can get more people thinking about it, is they will talk about the great Starbucks with someone buying a coffee and it goes on for hours or for 200 customers and it's awesome.

I love that they tell these stories but it's always a story that's buried 9 pages deep. It's always a story that's just a feel good story that they give to some junior journalist as an afterthought and personally, it's driving me crazy that that's an afterthought. It drives me nuts that the power of this movement is nothing but a page 9 type of article and on top of that they give no credit. They talk about people buying coffee, you should feel good and that's it. So you get tens of thousands or even hundreds of thousands of people reading that article and they have nowhere to go, no way to come back to us or to the foundation. They have nowhere to go to take the next step.

Kindness is always this afterthought that it's never been something that should be an immediate part of your day on a daily basis. It's always something around Christmas or Thanksgiving and personally I can't handle it. I understand the power of this, so what's going on now is we're begging journalists and people who are talking about us to understand this is a 365/24/7 type of process. It's not something you do when people are looking or around the holidays because you feel you need to sleep at night. This is something that the world needs help each and every day. There are people around you that need help each and every day.

It's something that I personally believe can be one of the most powerful things on the face of this planet and not a single human being, not one of the 7.1 billion people has an excuse as to why they can't help someone next to them. There's no money involved. Make someone smile. Do something for a family member, a stranger or a neighbor. It doesn't matter what country you live in, how much money you have or how you were brought up, your ideals or religions, this is what thing that the world can be a part of on a day-to-day basis no matter who you are.

It takes away all human excuse, so we're getting more aggressive with having people talk more about that there is an organization, a movement and a way for people to get more involved so that we can move up that page 9 article to page 4, page 3 or the front page. To get it to the point where it's a constant reminder and something that becomes subconscious and it becomes a habit. That's the thing, we need it to become a habit on a day-to-day basis and it's not that way yet.

Robyn: Wow! I feel chills because I can relate to your energetics of what you're sharing. It's like for me, being in practice for 21 years with at least 8000 treatments, traveled the world and seeing so much unnecessary suffering. It's like we want this idea of self-care to be like… it's a way of life it's not just something we do once in a while. This is one of our taglines that we say… it's a way of life. It's the true healthcare and to know that repetition and habit you talked about, that also in this framework of self-care it is so key and important that we Pay It Forward everyday.

That is part of human nature is that we're part of community. We are here to help each other, everybody no matter what your economic needs, needs a hand now and then. Everybody. I'm just always so struck when I travel and that's where I see the Pay It Forward. It happens everyday but I see so many things happen to Pay It Forward when I'm on a plane or getting lost in traffic. It's something that again doesn't have to be when I'm traveling, I'm just saying that through this exploration of our self-care movement and as we've built towards this month, and it's not like we're saying this is the only month to Pay It Forward, we're just saying now that you've regained your sense of self and you've taken back this most important decision of your life to practice self-care in everyday life, it's apiece of self-care, this gratitude piece and paying it forward.

I hear you and feel your energetics around this big time.

Charley: We just have to keep pushing.

Robyn: We know and we know the big why. Again, we know this message is so huge and will save so many lives. There are a lot of unnecessary suffering will not happen, prevention reverse disease and still this act of paying it forward is huge. It's like you talking about the story of this woman that happened 30 years earlier. It's like she's there right now having that experience and how that has brought such joy to her physiology and how that has shifted her from the inside out and to Pay It Forward.

Charley: Absolutely.

Kevin: In my work with synergy psychology I talk a lot about frequency and vibration and how that interacts with the physical body. We've structured this Self-Care Revolution™ that gratitude and paying it forward emerge out of this sense of well-being from taking care of the self. It is a natural loop back around to want to give to others when we are feeling energized and alive. I think that we can certainly hear that passion in your voice as you're talking about making this an everyday occurrence instead of every 30 years.

Charley: Yes. Not only do we believe that it can be an everyday occurrence, but I believe it can be something that goes down in history and something we talk about for hundreds of years, something that's one of the biggest things on the face of the planet. I believe that, because it's something that can infiltrate day to day life of everything. If you think of it you can be part of it. It can be part of religion or not. It can be part of a corporation or part of your neighborhood, your community, your city, your state, your school, your individual, your family, anything. Any single group, thing or living being it can infiltrate.

It can infiltrate and make every aspect of life around 207 + countries. It can infiltrate everyday life in every country however that country lives and however they are or whoever they are. It can be a part of lifting the fabric of that society up no matter how low they are, how war torn they are or how bad they are, how wealthy they are or how poor they are. I believe it's the thing. It feels right. It's that thing that feels so right that I've yet to have someone come up to us and say this isn't going to work, this can't work or this is not the right way. It's such a simple thing. There's nothing for us.

Kevin: It is interesting how it emerges from you like the first person that said okay I'm going to buy someone else's coffee. It's definitely these things that naturally emerge, but I love the fact that on your website and blog you have some suggestions. I'm looking at one of the Christmas suggestions about being a designated driver and going to a nursing home. Do you have more of those that you can share with us here?

Charley: There are hundreds. The app has a daily suggestion of making someone smile, hugging someone there are tons.

Kevin: That's awesome. Once you look at this list, it goes from donating blood to putting change in a parking meter. We've talked about those in our video about this month. Going to a soup kitchen or donating your time. Those are some of the bigger things but I think it's nice for people to know that really this is an instantaneous decision you can make like the flower or leaving a flower on a co-workers desk, I like that.

Charley: That's a fun one.

Robyn: I love what our speaker said last week when she was talking about entitlement ends basically when gratitude begins. To say the same thing with Pay It Forward, the action of paying it forward and how that shifts. When you think about the epidemic of depression and people being victim of their life circumstances. When you start paying it forward and doing good for others, that can majorly shift you from the inside out, from your cells to your organs and to your being-ness. It's powerful.

Kevin: You have another simple concept but I'd like you to share a little about this. The idea of being pro-kindness as opposed to anti-bullying that's currently going on in schools right now.

Charley: This is a heated subject. When I was a kid as most people were kids, when our parents told us not to do something what did we want to do? We wanted that cookie. We wanted to wear that. We wanted to do everything our parents told us not to do. Mother Theresa would go to a pro-peace rally but not an anti-war rally. Every school nowadays because of all this bullying and I wish we could just stop talking about it, because it just makes things worse.

So celebrities go into these schools and we have hundreds of millions of dollars behind anti-bullying. It's part of every school curriculum now, every district and all these people walk in doing this one-time assembly and say don't do this or that. Don't... and we continue to wonder why year after year it gets worse. We're having them focus on nothing but what they shouldn't do and look who gets attention, the bad kids. The negative stuff gets the attention. The, what they shouldn't do gets the attention. Psychologically it messes with them and it makes more people become what they shouldn't be.

I'm a huge believer in walking into a school like we do and giving the kids something to build from not to tear down, something good to talk about, something good to do rather than telling them everything they shouldn't do. These teachers unfortunately are locked in to what their district does or what the principal says. So we have teachers from all over the world come to us and say we have anti-bully but I'm much more of a fan of what you all are doing, can we purchase some bracelets and they'll just start it in their classrooms.

Then the next thing you know it goes to the grade level and then to the entire school. The anti-bullying thing, when you walk into a school and tell them what they shouldn't do, it only includes those students you're talking about. Everyone leaves there thinking, gosh I can't do this or that and it's such a negative feeling. When you bring Pay It Forward, pro-kindness and bracelets to the schools it spreads and goes not only from the school to the teaches but those bracelets make their way to the families when they get home, to the community when they get out and evolve to other schools.

Wouldn't you rather have something that's positive that spreads, rather than something negative, let's talk about everything we shouldn't do and stays within the school? That doesn't make sense to me, yet because we have a train and all this money, effort and momentum behind anti-bully and because we as adults don't want to say we're wrong and we want to just keep cramming this down because that's what we thought would work six years ago, we're just going to keep doing it. And year after year we're going to keep doing the same things. We need hindsight because doing the same things over and over expecting different results is the definition of insanity.

Yet, year after year we do the same stuff, spend the same money on the same things with the same anti-bully programs and yet every newscast has another kid committing suicide, another one getting bullied and we just sit there and say how disgusting it is. Oh, let's do anti-bully? No, let's focus on something we can build on rather than stop everything and tearing things down. It drives me crazy and it doesn't work!

Kevin: I know we're looking at all these different ways to communicate now, like you mentioned Facebook and Twitter and those are being used for that negative purpose to harass or, because you are so available to these levels of communication, but just the simple concept of... last week we did that by turning it around with a little gratitude text and that was such a powerful thing. We did these texts when we were doing the interview and got messages back immediately from people.

To think of this in a way of instead of sharing on your Facebook post what you had for lunch, saying something nice to some specific people that are friends on Facebook.

Charley: Yeah, don't even get me started on Facebook.

Robyn: I'm going to comment on what you shared, Charley, that makes me think of the war against cancer, against poverty, against you name it and what we're doing is simply perpetuating the against rather than saying... what we're doing with the Self-Care Revolution™ is saying these are the great choices you have in terms of whole, organic, non-GMO foods. These are the choices you have instead of exercising being so difficult, painful and to be avoided it can be just a 10 minute something five times a week, that's better than not at all. So again, what are we for not what are we against.

I hear what you're saying and I love your solution. I have a 12 and 14 year olds and I hear of the bullying happening in their school and I would love to see this proactivity. Just being proactive and doing something with this mindset and I love that this is part of your mission. It's part of mine and Kevin's as well and many of us that are part of the Self-Care Revolution™, quite a few around the globe as well as those listening that say yes I'm here to learn more and deepen my awareness of what I am for, to have excellent, optimal and sustainable health.

I feel that for so many people that aren't participating in society or being of service, there are excuses. They don't have energy. They can't walk. The more that this message is shared and the more people get this into their system that this is a way of life, a 365/24/7 concept almost like breathing air, it should be natural, we're here to participate and contribute, to Pay It Forward and to receive.

Charley: We should find a way to become better mentally, physically or with our habits each day. I know that's so cliché and I have a tough time with the self-help stuff and everything, but we really should, especially as adults. I play basketball and I sit there and watch the guys I play ball with that are 40-50 and it's getting through life, waking up, going to work and playing a little ball or working out once in a while. It's not about still reading. They think their education is over it was back in college and it's not about reading different topics to expand your viewpoint of world topics. It's mentally your habits.

It's the same guys staying the same weight, doing the same things, becoming the same people and not doing anything different. Why else would we want to wake up in the morning? Why wouldn't we want to do something that's going to make us a tiny happier, a bit smarter, wiser, a tiny anything.

Kevin: It does go to how powerful we are as individuals and how we forget that. This culture generally promotes the wealth, the physical and the ways of how we can have more things and I think just a small piece of this, tip a server 50% instead of 15%, that's so simple. I started the practice of pre-tipping before the service happens and integrity with the process that it's not something I'm paying you for just as you're giving me service. That really changed my perspective and people think that's weird but it's one of those things you can do.

Charley: I love it.

Kevin: It's fun and it becomes a fun part of life and I hear that in your voice, making this a fun habit of gee, I'm getting in my car and heading out, what Pay It Forward thing can I do today? Or how many I can do, maybe that could be your challenge in the course of an average day.

Charley: Absolutely.

Kevin: You mentioned the app. Can we direct people to a place on your website where they can download this?

Charley: They can go to the same website I mentioned earlier. There's a tab at the top for app. Right now, in my opinion, it's a good app but simple. It's a simple app of a daily suggestion. You can see the daily suggestion. It could be something you can do that day or you could choose to do whatever you want. It shows you across the world where people have dropped pens and done deeds across the world. There isn't much to it, but for all the listeners we will have something... it will be amazing, during the second quarter of 2014. That app right now is a great reminder to see on your phone or iPad or tablet, to see in the morning with a push notification to give you an idea or suggestion.

If it works it works and if it doesn't it doesn't.

Robyn: It's a free app for people.

Charley: Right now it's $.99.

Robyn: That's perfect. We'll do our best to support this movement by getting this interview out to as many people as possible. Sometimes I think people have to hear your perspective. It's around this time where people say I love this time, I love Thanksgiving it's my favorite holiday because it's all about giving and the whole time brings this up, but there are a lot of negativity that shows up around the season as well. Put it into a new perspective.

The app is super-useful and we can use them in our busy lives today as reminders until it becomes a habit. You always want to be giving and paying something forward to someone, paying that kindness forward.

Charley: Absolutely.

Robyn: This all ties in with our message that we're all about with this movement. For everyone listening, how I found Charley is as we were going into our final money of this first year of the Self-Care Revolution™ series I thought, if I'm going to Google Pay It Forward I wonder what will come up first. I found Charley, and I also found out about the movie and I thought I should go back to the movie. It did okay but not great. Can you talk about why you think that happened? Give us some insight into that.

Charley: When we got serious about this movement in 2011 and decided to dedicate all our time to it, the first thing you look towards is the book, which Katherine is awesome and she's on the board of our Foundation. She's always there when we need her. Then you look to the movie and there's almost nothing more powerful than a movie with tens of thousands of eyeballs seeing that movie. People reached out to Helen Hunt and Kevin Spacey in the movie before and didn't receive anything. We started digging deeper and you get the true story.

Financially I wouldn't say it was a disaster but I wouldn't say it was a moneymaker for Warner Brothers. I've heard stories of the actors not really agreeing on the direction of the movie. The critics from what I've seen and heard tore the actors apart. So to them it was a job. They enjoyed the movie and the movement, but it wasn't the highlight of their career or something they could look back on and say, people thought I did a good job and the movie made a ton of money. So they could have shied away from it.

Getting in touch with them is next to impossible. I've never seen any of them talk about it. They've all moved on and that's not a problem, I just thought that with that movie, with Warner Brothers, it would be a great thing that would create more momentum to see if we can work something out. The only thing I've seen is that that movie has shown more in the past few years. They can sense it. They have smart people working for them. They see how many people are talking about Pay It Forward. That movie is on all the time and I'm assuming they've recouped the money they didn't make initially.

I will say that in 2012, Kevin Spacey has the old Vick Theater in London and we were over there touring around and doing some talks and speaking to some schools, and we created enough buzz that he started seeing what was going on. I don't remember who knew his assistant or something, but we asked if we did a screening and he allowed us to have his theater for free for one night and to play Pay It Forward. We brought a couple hundred people there to watch the movie and did some Q&A after. He knows what we're up to but it's 13 years ago and it wasn't the highlight of their career so they don't talk about it much.

Robyn: That's fascinating. I think it's great that you're keeping this legacy alive in all the ways you're doing this. I commend you and think it's fantastic. Again, I love how this has enlivened the Pay It Forward spirit in me, in our center and especially in our revolution. It has been great to hear your perspective of it.

I want to mention too that we started a non-profit, the Santa Fe Soul Foundation several years ago in 2005/2006 and the purpose of it is to offer financial support to people that are challenged in that way to have access to complementary alternative healthcare, because basically what's available is Medicaid, prescription drugs and not much of what we in the complementary world offer, which is helping people to get back to nature and back to healthy foods and all that.

The point is we decided as we gave grants, whether it was $250, $500 or $1000 to people who qualified that we said we would like you to Pay It Forward and we partnered with 20 other non-profits. It was neat how that came up. I remember the day and the woman who, as we were saying we don't just want to give away free healthcare to people in need, how do we have that person not just take it and how do they then Pay It Forward. This is the message to of the Self-Care Revolution™ is that we make these shifts in our lives and we know that we have this bounty, abundance and great energy to share, regardless of our health.

We can do that of course, but it seems to be true that as we've seen people go through this 12 month series, as they feel better you're on fire and you want to help. Your next career, next step in life, your passion, your purpose has been realized through a transformation of your own health.

I'm thinking about Terry Wahls, who we interviewed in November for gratitude. She's a medical doctor who was diagnosed with MS and now she's returned herself to health as much as possible. She's writing a book and is speaking everywhere. She is paying it forward in a big way to say you know what there are alternatives to drugs in this case. I just want to say with all the ways in which we can Pay It Forward are endless.

Like you said Charley, bringing it into our businesses, our school, our communities and even in our relationships.

Charley: Day to day life.

Kevin: Making it a habit. I think that's important; is there any final words you'd like to share with the audience today?

Charley: Not really. I enjoy these interviews because they get a different opinion and they get to see that there's more substance to this than just buying someone's coffee. There's a global movement and so many ways for them to contact us and get involved, their families but I'm biased. I love this movement. I'm very cynical and like the Devil's advocate for so many things in this world and I've tried to be that say way with Pay It Forward just so I'm not thinking this the wrong way. It's so simple and anyone listening can get involved this very second.

Robyn: That's awesome. You must be like 33 years old.

Charley: Yes.

Robyn: You're young. The future looks wonderful with you being at the core of this message and all the people that care to be part of this ripple of change project that you've started. It's fantastic.

Charley: Thank you for having me and helping me spread the message.

Robyn: Thank you so much. Absolutely. What does a self-care day look like for you?

Charley: A day-to-day process.

Robyn: How you take care of yourself and how you keep this movement alive and well.

Charley: Probably all that you're doing. I work out everyday, lots of basketball, cardio and lifting. I'm also experimenting with organic foods and cutting much out of my diet. It's amazing what we put into our bodies that we think is good. I watch the diet, work out and read a lot to get as much info into my head as I can.

Robyn: We have a live event coming in June 2014, our 2nd Annual Self-Care Lifestyle Bliss event, it would be great to have you here live with us and to share your story, your journey and getting these bracelets out to 122 countries that's fantastic.

Charley: That'd be great.

Robyn: Thanks again for being with us. For all of you, happy holidays in whatever way you're celebrating. We love you and send our blessings. Take care.

[End of Interview]

MARCIA WIEDER

DreamUniversity.com | CEO/Founder Of Dream University, Author, Columnist, And Speaker

MEANING: THE ELIXIR OF LIFE OR THE MEANING OF LIFE

[These statements have not been evaluated by the Food and Drug Administration. The information on this audiocast is not intended to diagnose, treat, cure, or prevent any disease.]

Robyn: Hello everyone and welcome to month 12 of the Self-Care Revolution™. This is quite a special and extraordinary day, the last day of 2013, our first year of the Self-Care Revolution™. I want to thank all of you that have been with us since the very beginning. As you know, we started out with Marcia Wieder and we are ending our series with the amazing Marcia Wieder. We're so excited. Thank you for being here, Marcia.

Marcia: I'm thrilled and honored. Thank you.

Robyn: For all of you, if you happen to be listening for the first time, my name is Robyn Benson. I'm a Doctor of Oriental Medicine. I'm the founder of Santa Fe Soul Health and Healing Center. I just want to say it has been such an honor and a privilege and a year of extraordinary growth to be facilitating this Self-Care Revolution™. It's totally revolutionized my life in many ways. We have so much in store for next year, so just stay tuned because we have a lot we want to share with you from this full-year series. And my wonderful co-host is here.

Kevin: Kevin Snow, Intuitive Counselor, I've just been amazed by this wild revolutionary ride that we've had this year and so grateful to be part of this last day of this year's Self-Care Revolution™ and so grateful to have Marcia to begin this process of going after our dreams and boy we sure have this year. Thank you so much, Marcia.

Marcia: I'm actually blown away by what you guys have created. It's one thing to host a one-time teleseminar and a huge undertaking to do it over a month. I can't imagine even a part of me knows what it took to do it for an entire year with the caliber of the speakers, the quality of the content and the beautiful intention behind this entire revolution. You guys really, really deserve to be acknowledged and appreciated. I'm just thankful that I got to be there in the beginning when you were still finding your voices as interviewers and here we are a year later at the end of the year just bringing it all to culmination. Thanks for doing this. Yeah to you guys!

Robyn: Thank you, Marcia. Also, you were one of our keynote speakers at our live event in June. That was such a great experience to have you here at our center and people loved you. You obviously were one of the favorites and people are going to be following you this year to your live event in April.

Marcia: Yes! I'm excited that you and Kevin both and hundreds of people will be out for the Wealthy Visionary Conference in L.A. in April. I'm really excited because, as a speaker, sometimes I just kind of drop in and touch people's hearts; maybe say something that awakens them. It's so different when I get to see people months or years later to really hear that what we've brought to them has touched, inspired and impacted their lives in some way. I'm excited about deepening our friendships and continuing this revolution of awakening.

Robyn: We're also excited that we're sharing this interview time with you with Harmony West, one of our beloved Self-Care coaches.

Harmony: Thanks, Robyn. Marcia, we all learned so much from you at the Bliss Weekend, so I'm totally excited.

Marcia: Well, Harmony, I'm so glad that you spoke up and I got to say hi to you, as well. I'm looking forward to seeing you again.

Harmony: Ditto.

Robyn: So for all of you who are joining us for the first time with Marcia, Marcia Wieder is the CEO and founder of Dream University. With over 20 years of writing, coaching, training and speaking experience, her inspiring message has touched audiences from 70 to 70,000 at companies such as AT&T, Gap and American Express. Whether teaching at Stanford Business School, executives in China or Girl Scout camps, Marcia's powerful message impacts audiences worldwide.

Appearing several times on 'Oprah', the 'Today Show' and in her own PBS TV special, Marcia is a bestselling author who has written 14 books dedicated to achieving dreams. Recently succeeding, in spite of everything, named No. 1 in Amazon in 10 categories. I could just go on and on about the things you do. Marcia is a fabulous coach and I just have to say that I've been very fortunate this year to be in one of her mastermind groups. It's been a great experience. It certainly has stretched me. It's really helped me with this vision.

The Self-Care Revolution™ is a big vision I would have to say of many of us. As you know, we have attracted almost 120 speakers who have said yes to this Revolution. Knowing that this is a time of extraordinary change, we know this is the solution. Self-Care is the true health care. It is the solution to these sad situations we're seeing in our healthcare system. We're just asking everyone to make this commitment to be their own healthcare advocate, their own self-care advocate, knowing that you do not have to experience the suffering that so many do. Our goal, Kevin, do you want to say it? The big bodacious vision is?

Kevin: To connect and touch a billion lives.

Robyn: To prevent and reverse disease. Why not have a fun, fulfilled, engaged life and live your passions, live your visions, as Marcia says so well and shares with us. Marcia, I'm looking at our very first book. We have created a book for each month and, of course, Marcia, we have your whole transcript of that call one year ago. This is the very end of this year as we go into next year and you said, "It's a great time for us all to be focusing on our vision for the next year and kind of forget resolutions of what you want to let go of and get rid of and, instead, let's focus on your dreams and how you want your life to be." I love that.

Marcia: You know it's so funny, has it really been a year. It's like I just said that yesterday. I don't know. The older I get, the faster it goes by. When we focus on resolutions, typically, we're looking at what we want to get rid of. I want to lose weight. I want to quit smoking. I want to stop something. Energetically, it's always more powerful to move toward what we want then it is to move away from something.

For me, a dream really speaks to what is it you truly want, what is it that really matters to you, how do you want your life to be, what's really important to you. So one of my New Year's Eve rituals for the last 20 years has been to sit down and to write out what my dreams are for the next year. I often forget about the list and then the following New Year's Eve I'm pulling out the list (other people have said this, as well) and I'm always kind of amazed and tickled at how many things actually were accomplished and how many of the things I've not only accomplished, but even went beyond what I could imagine.

Then there are the ones that are on the list year in year out that don't happen. Now I've started actually dumping those because I feel if they're lingering they're kind of sucking my energy and I'm forever talking about it and if it really mattered to me I would do something about it. So I love this idea of focusing on what we want, what we want to create, how we want the next year to be as opposed to what we're resolving not to do or what we want to get rid of.

Robyn: I love that. That is a great way as we enter this New Year. We've got three of us, so we've got lots of great questions for you. We want to hear about this dream. Since you're known as the CEO of Dream University and this has been a big message, you work with some of the top companies, just any more you want to say. This has been kind of a tumultuous year for so many. You use this word a lot, 'a game-changer' year. Any more insights before we go into your new content in your book that you might want to share with all of us?

Marcia: One of the things is we could look back over a period of our life and there are always ups and downs, there is always this tumultuous timing. I don't know if it's the Internet and ease and the accessibility of information that makes it seem like it's so much more, you know more tsunamis, earthquakes and more terrible things happening, but also more wonderful, wondrous, extraordinary things happen. I've been practicing this concept recently that I call Everyday Enlightenment, which is to spend more time every day in the light connected to my dreams, my hopes and my desires; less time in the dark being hijacked by my fears and doubts, other people's fears and doubts and the news, ultimately, trying to live a life of virtue.

I think the highest virtue is a life of integrity and I think a life of integrity is more time in the light and less time in the dark. So I think this daily practice and maybe, if you're able to, adapting this belief that I have, which is it's never been a better or more important time for us to achieve our dreams or to pursue what matters to us. It's just now. I encourage people not to look in their checking account, not to look at the news and not to look at the stock market to decide whether or not a dream matters to you, but to go into your heart to find what really matters to you, to stand as strong as you're able to and to share the dream with other likeminded kindred spirits, people who are a part of revolutionary thinking and living who are committed to uplifting the planet.

As each of us says yes to what's in our heart and has the courage to step out, not because there are promises and guarantees or assurances, but rather because something matters to us, then each of us is contributing to the healing and the transformation of the planet, which is the bigger dream that I think we all share. Certainly in the Self-Care Revolution™, certainly any of us that are on a path of consciousness, we know that our thinking and our mindset, what's coming out of our month and certainly what we're doing, is contributing to the healing and the uplifting of the planet. So I want to say go for your dreams.

Harmony: You are so blessed inspiring. Talk about everyday enlightenment. I mean, basically, what you're doing is helping us ground enlightenment, Marcia, in the every day.

Marcia: Exactly. I also think it's important for us to know that we each matter. I think it can feel so overwhelming and so many things can feel like they are out of control. One of the things that listeners to this call can do if you want a little free gift from me, I put together something called The 12 Ways to be a 21st Century Visionary kit. If you just go to my website www.dreamuniversity.com, you can opt-in. It's a one-page PDF and a radio interview. The number one thing I think we can do to live more visionary, to live more of this everyday enlightenment, is to get comfortable with uncertainty.

The reality of it is we do live in uncertain times. That is what life is about. So, again, it's not about these guarantees that so many of us want, the little control freak that each of us inside of us, but the ability to get comfortable with uncertainty so we can dance with life, so we can be malleable, so when challenging, difficult and even painful things or scary things happen, we remember that we have the capacity to center ourselves, that we remember there are the practical things we can do like breathing and opening our heart and the spiritual things we can do.

I heard this wonderful song lyric this weekend, 'why worry when you can pray'. Isn't that amazing? It's just like the best lyric, why worry when you can pray. If we can remember during these challenging and not so challenging times that we actually do have a say in how our life goes and how our days unfold, then I think we can come back to feeling spiritual wholly and at a very simple level empowered.

Harmony: That sounds like a good segue into you being able to start talking to us about the new ideas that you're bringing forward about meaning and this being the elixir of life.

Marcia: Yes, it's a very exciting thing to recreate yourself. As you said, I've written 14 books, 30 years of my life talking to people about making their dreams come true and the dream that I've heard people talk about that's most important and that they talk about most often is we want to know that our life matters. We want to know that our life has meaning. After three years of being on a passion quest, taking a period of time of saying no thank you to what was no longer true for me, emptying, slowing down and deepening while I was still running my business, while I still had to pay my bills. It wasn't like I checked out of life, but I really shifted into a different gear sensing there was something else that wanted to come through and low and behold there it was.

I feel like this next 30 years of my life or however long it's meant to be, I feel like this new message is as significant for me as dreaming was 30 years ago. It was dreaming and now it's meaning. We hear a lot of people talking about purpose and I talk about purpose, as well. Without knowing what your purpose is, we sometimes climb to the top of the mountain to discover it's the wrong mountain. Well, what I started really realizing about meaning is that we are meaning-making machines. We give everything that happens meaning, but typically we give it a negative meaning or a negative expectation. We feel or imagine the worst and yet we know that living a meaningful life is tied directly into fulfillment.

If we look at kind of the cost of no meaning vs. the chaos, especially within the context of what you guys are all about, the Self-Care Revolution™, a life of no meaning is painful. I think it brings up fear and often confusion, what am I doing with my life or the fear of running out of time and money and not having done something meaningful with my life. I think people who are mired in loss of meaning feel a sense of emptiness. Maybe they're aging faster. They and we (I can talk about this as myself) feel lonely or sometimes worthless or unfulfilled, insignificant. I mean the list goes on and on.

If we contrast that with a meaningful life, when I'm connected to what matters to me, I feel like I've got a reason in my life. I feel like I have self-esteem. I feel more fulfilled. I have more faith and gratitude. I feel like I'm making a contribution. I feel more optimistic. I stop aging. I look and feel healthier and younger.

So I'm really in this exploration around meaning and I know that our life has meaning, yet the studying of it, the writing about it, the talking about it, has been a very, very challenging process, to my surprise and, hopefully, not to my demise. I'll tell you one reason why and then I'm happy to go wherever you want to go with this.

Oh, this is so vulnerable. I so don't even want to say it, but I will anyway. I wasn't ready that in writing about meaning I would have to come face to face with all the places in my life that feel meaningless.

It's like oh, I so don't want to feel that. I want to skip right to the second half of the book where I give you all the prescriptions. I want to give you the meaning map. I want to give you the meaning quotient and the life score card. It's got all of these prescriptions and these tools. I wanted to skip the first half, but the first half is I thought what don't I want to write? What don't I want to say?

I don't want to say that I'm a 57-year-old single woman who has no children, where most of my friends are couples and have families, so that I often feel lonely and alone. What I don't want to say is that I judge myself for feeling this way. On one hand I see myself as beautiful, healthy, wealthy, loved and adored. I have so much reason to really be so grateful for my life, but it's the judgment of feeling meaningless that makes it even feel worse.

So here I just got back from the Galapagos Islands. I'm on a 100-foot yacht with 14 people, so many people's dream and on their bucket list, and what I notice is that most of the people on the boat are drinking for lunch and dinner. I don't really judge it. I'm just not a drinker so I didn't feel that I could join into the conversation. I was on this boat and I didn't feel like I had one meaningful conversation with another person and was just feeling worse and worse about myself.

I was able to take a step back and say okay, this is what needs to be written. That no matter where we are in life, all of us at different times are faced with this dark side of feeling inadequate, less than, insufficient, something was wrong and then something is wrong that something was wrong. It just kind of sets off the spiral and I think when I'm with friends, when I'm with circles of friends and colleagues, what we're talking about is the longing for more meaning. What we're hungry for is to know that we're using our lives in service to something good.

I also am hearing more and more as we're getting older this sense of wanting to create a legacy. To know that my contribution was not just my children or even a successful business, but that I'm actually making a contribution in an area that's meaningful which will then touch and impact other people's lives, as well.

So, anyway, that was a big, long answer. We can break it down and we can go wherever you want to with this, but I can tell you it hasn't been an easy topic. Once I finally got clear that this is what I've been asked to do and to write about right now, it hasn't all been a bowl of cherries. That's just my honest revealing of my relationship to meaning right now.

Kevin: That was really beautiful.

Robyn: Speaking of legacy, what a legacy with all the books that you've written and all the people you've coached. Marcia, you are amazing. Speaking of legacy, you're going to be speaking at a conference coming up next month. Could you speak about that a little bit, the Legacy Conference?

Marcia: It's not my event. I'm a speaker at it. It's just really a lot of colleagues and friends coming together wanting to contribute to one of our sweet sisters and one of my closest friends Cynthia Kersey with the Unstoppable Foundation. It's really talking about contribution and service and doing what's meaningful for you in a way that really can contribute and help other people.

Robyn: And that's meaningful, all the work she's doing to build schools.

Marcia: Oh, yeah. You know I kept asking myself what's meaningful, but you just said it. I love that. Where does meaning come from? On one hand what's meaningful is what matters to you, as an individual what matters to you. So I'm on the board of the Make a Wish Foundation. I'm on Cynthia's board. We get in touch with what matters to us and, hopefully, that's the place where we can contribute.

The other thing that seems to be meaningful for us is a sense of belonging and connection. Certainly, Brené Brown talks about this in her wonderful TED talk. I thought it was very interesting. As part of my research and meaning, I went back and re-watched that talk and heard something I hadn't heard the first time. She talked about that when we have a low self-worth, we often don't ever feel that we belonged. It's an interesting thing because it's kind of a vicious cycle. If I have a low self-worth and I feel like I don't belong, well then I feel like I'm living a meaningless life which then takes me back to feeling worthless or less than. It can be this really vicious cycle.

Meaning comes from doing what matters to you, but meaning also comes by belonging to something, so when we can belong to something that's meaningful. Also, there's a tremendous amount of research in the health fields coming out now that shows meaning distinct from happiness, that happiness often sets people up for a sense that something is missing. The health symptoms or health challenges we often see with people who are suffering with chronic illness are some of the same disease symptoms that are showing up for people who talk about that they're in search of happiness. This is just shocking.

The distinction between happiness and meaning is happiness we tend to focus more on ourselves. What do I need in order to feel happy? Meaning is we tend to focus on something outside of ourselves like making a contribution or being part of something that's bigger than ourselves.

I'll just throw this in real quickly. There was also a study just recently in August of this year in the Harvard Business Review. Oh, here, this is exactly what I was talking about. "People who report that they are missing a sense of meaning in their lives are less likely to exhibit the chronic stress response associated with life-threatening diseases like heart disease and cancers that do still show up when people are talking about the pursuit of happiness."

It's amazing that that pursuit of happiness can still trigger heart disease and some of those other kinds of cancers that we're seeing. Happiness is also more equated with disappointment then meaning. I mean it's just fascinating to me. I don't even really understand it yet. I'm still in the like what?

Kevin: I think that definitely brings up a good point, too, Marcia. The thing you have that is propelling you in this direction is this curiosity.

Marcia: I love that. Thank you for saying that. Also, I will tell you it's my own longing for meaning. I started researching one of the competing books, because right now I'm writing a book on meaning, and there's not been much specifically around meaning since Viktor Frankl's *Man's Search for Meaning*, which he wrote in a holocaust in a concentration camp. Yet it's a big conversation. There's a lot of dialogue.

I guess what I would say is your life has meaning. You are here for a noble purpose and what there is to do is to discover it. I don't hold it that it's the Holy Grail that your lifelong pursuit is to discover what's meaningful for you, but rather how do you make every moment or every day a meaningful experience. It is a reframe and there is a shifting in the lens of our perception and, of course, there is a mindset. We can point to well, it's about gratitude and it's about appreciation, but first I think we have to get really conscious about what is meaningful for us. I think a lot of us don't even know what that is.

It's so funny. My editor said to me well, what do you mean by meaning? She was like I'm not really sure what that means. I said well, it's everywhere. I can joke. I said remember the move 'The Gods Must Be Crazy'? A Coke bottle falls out of the sky and the village has never seen one. They have no history and they have no story and, therefore, it doesn't mean anything. Now, we make up meaning, so I can either make it up to mean that it's a very hip brand and Coke is kind of cool or it's a toxic beverage to boycott. I can give it meaning.

What I think a lot of us have forgotten is that we live every minute of our life with meaning. Let me paint you a little picture. My alarm clock goes off, which means I'm either on time or I'm late. I jump into the shower and I use all these products that are probably overpriced, which means if I smell a certain way I'll be more attractive or successful. I prepare an organic breakfast while feeding my dogs' organic food because it might actually in real life mean it's better for them.

You know that I dress and I accessorize believing that how I look means something about who I am. I get in my car and I follow the signs that are going to get me to work on time, but if I make a wrong turn or my karma is bad that day, I'm not going to find a parking spot. Throughout the entire day I'm assigning meaning all the way until my head hits the pillow and even then the book that's lying next to my bed is *The Meaning of My Dreams*.

We assign meaning to everything based on our conditioning, which actually renders it meaningless at a certain level. So if we can arbitrarily attach meaning based on some history or some belief, what are the practices we can put in place to create a much more meaningful existence every day, which will then give us more joy, more fulfillment, and more resource. That's really the message that I'm feeling called to write about right now as I figure it out for myself.

Kevin: That's so important because what you're doing is you're essentially redirecting us from an exterior meaning or a meaning that's being placed on us by maybe the media or friends or family and you're redirecting us to this internal compass that is saying this is what's meaningful to us and helping us to do that. Some of the things you talked about in our original conversation were how to get over some of these basic obstacles. One of the things I really loved was the ability to say no and how to say no to the things that no longer have powerful meaning.

Marcia: I thank you for that punctuation and so clearly, Kevin. Where that ties into this message, the critical point is meaning is a choice, so as we learn how to make conscious choices based on what's important to us, including saying no thank you or saying yes, getting clear about discernment, what needs to be in place for me to say yes. I don't always have a choice, but when I do have the choice let me choose what matters to me, what's meaningful to me and let me even choose how I'm seeing it, viewing it, interpreting it and, therefore, engaging with it.

For me, our Creator's greatest gift to humanity is that we have the ability to create. You can, we can, create a life based on what we value, based on what matters to us and even based on what makes us feel significant. So if out of this message people learn how to choose and create and ultimately live a meaningful life, I will die happy and fulfilled.

You know what I hear myself doing now? It's very funny, I'm making it illusive. Once I have this then I'll have meaning as opposed to wow, my life is already so meaningful and so rich and let me catch myself in the moment of judging and criticizing and belittling and all those things we do that bring up all those feelings of inadequacy or scarcity. Let me be in the practice. God, please hear my prayer. Let me be in the practice of catching myself in the act of doing something where I'm being less than my Divine self or less than the appreciator of the Divinity that of us have and allow me to course correct more quickly.

I think that's what enlightenment is, that we bounce back faster, that our reactions become less and that we look at (sounds so simple) the cup as being half full, but then that we're grateful and appreciate that we have something to drink at all.

Robyn: I think of this exploration of self-care and the correlation with meaning. I mean the ultimate self-care is when we are living a meaningful life. I can't help but think as we continue this discussion of "Nothing is either good or bad, only perception makes it so", Shakespeare's quote.

Marcia: Beautiful.

Robyn: I love it. It's just such a powerful one in this exploration of meaning, the perception piece and how we can really get ourselves in trouble in terms of what we perceive to be meaningful or not meaningful based on our own background or own life experiences. Can you talk a little bit about that?

Marcia: I just so love that because, for me, the converse is true, as well. One of the ways that I practice self-care is by appreciating life, by bringing meaning. Instead of lobbing meaning, I'm bringing meaning. What a way to heal and to nurture. You know life can really look like a black and white program of we're running that tape now, now we're running that program and life loses its texture, its color, its luster. In any moment I can take a breath and I can bring color in by connecting to what I care about, by connecting to what I love, by bringing what's meaningful to it.

I can be with my family at a holiday meal and be whiny, complaining, seeing everybody as their story or in a moment I can choose to see the Divinity in each person and be so grateful that I'm alive and assign the meaning that this is a holy moment where I'm gathered with people who may be Mashugana, crazy and drive me nuts, but they're my family and I love them, I adore them, I appreciate them and they're my greatest teachers. So in a moment something painful or meaningless can become so rich and so valuable.

That is self-care. I think self-care is the moment by moments, at the very least the day by day, but the moment by moment course correcting and practicing until it becomes the fiber of who we are and suddenly I notice I'm laughing more. I'm just more relaxed and my mind is quieter. The disease isn't coming because I'm actually resonating at a higher frequency of joy, of meaningful, of the sense of belonging. My old story of being inadequate or not belonging or having a low self-worth becomes lesser and lesser and eventually disappears as a conversation. So, for me, meaning is directly tied to self-care.

Harmony: That's so profound. I'm going to quote you on that.

Marcia: I'm going to listen to the replay of this and have good content for my book.

Robyn: The disease is not coming because I'm feeling more joy and meaning in my life. That is huge. That is really the message behind this Self-Care Revolution™ is that we don't have to go to that place by experiencing all these messages of self-care.

Marcia: And you know what, any one of us. I can be with a group of people and if they're whining and complaining, which we all go to, or gossiping, I can just join the conversation and then we stay at that low vibration. I can also say nothing and then I have a weird sense of not belonging because everybody is gossiping. I can walk away, but now I'm not part of the group or I can raise the conversation.

I can be meaningful. I can be the bright light. I can be the spark in that moment that brings another point of view of gratitude and appreciation and I've shifted a room full of 1,000 plus people by being the bright light and I maintain that each of us has that gift within us. Whether it's a one-on-one conversation with your spouse, your children, your parent, let's be the bright light, that's really it, and remind each other that we all have that Divinity within us.

Kevin: That's such a perfect link to finish off our conversation on paying it forward because that is paying it forward. That is the definition that you just gave us there of being the light, being the one that basically takes a situation that we see every day, situations that are judgmental and lower energy and move them to this higher frequency of light.

Robyn: Thank you, Kevin, for mentioning. This 12th month of our first year of the Self-Care Revolution™ Series is all about paying it forward. What a perfect message you're sharing with us, Marcia, about that. When you feel more meaning deep in your life and in your day-to-day activities it's contagious, that vibration that you're speaking about. It's that bright light that you're sharing with the world.

Marcia: And it gives us more. You know the conversation around scarcity then goes away. It's the end of the year. I'm tithing. I'm making my donations. We have a big event coming up. If people want to know about it it's called the Wealthy Visionary Conference, just go to WealthyVisionary.com. We'll be tithing at this event back to the educational system to teach our future generation of children to dream meaningful dreams. So if you're listening to this and you have a dream and you're wanting to reach more people and have greater impact, if you're wanting to learn how to monetize your dream and you're wanting to spend four days with me, the full ticket price is $1,997. It's almost $2,000.

It will say on the registration page we have 200 tickets left. We actually only have 70 tickets, but we left up our Early Bird Special a little longer for your people so people who want to come can come for $697. That's only going to be up for a few more days, so if you're wanting to spend four days with me being laser coached learning how to share your big dream and be in a room with 500 people -- the room only holds 500 and we've sold 430 tickets -- our fabulous host will be there, Robyn will be there, Kevin will be there, Harmony will be there and I will be there. You can sign up today for $697, just go to WealthyVisionary.com.

This is not a multi-speaker event with a lot of people selling you stuff. This is an in-depth workshop where I'm going to take you to the depth of your soul, help you open to a much bigger vision and help you leave with the very practical tools and brilliant shortcuts so you can bring your vision to the world. The theme is the conference is Bridging Money and Meaning, so if you've got something and you want to bring it out to the world and you want to monetize it so you can become more generous, have more ability to be philanthropic, *Pay It Forward* and help other people, come be in a room full of people who share your vision.

Whether you're passionate or what matters to you is the environment or education, our youth or single moms, food and, of course, health and making the world a healthier place, you are going to have an opportunity to be with extraordinary people. If you do make it to the event, please come over and seek me out. Let me know that you've heard about this on the Self-Care Revolution™. Those of you that met me, obviously, while I was in Santa Fe, I look forward to playing with you guys. I will be very accessible and very available throughout the entire four days of the event.

So if you're serious about making this the best year of your life and you've got a dream or you're even in search of a new dream and you want to find some extraordinary people that you can collaborate with, take a look at WealthyVisionary.com and if it's a good fit for you grab one of the Early Bird spots before that price goes up to the full $1,997 or before the program sells out.

Kevin: We're excited to be there.

Marcia: I loved being at the Santa Fe Soul Center and doing my session with Kevin and, of course, getting healing with Robyn and so many extraordinary beings and beautiful souls and kindred spirits. So, for me, we'll have a quality of a reunion times 500. Kevin, I want you to know that my prayers are with you and your family during this holiday time as you're dealing. I know that people will be listening to the replays throughout the entire year, but we're live right now and I want you, personally, to know that I'm sending you tremendous love and healing prayers for your mom. I just am sending you so much love and light during this challenging time.

Kevin: Thank you so much. I truly appreciate that and she does, as well, as she goes through this process that we are talking about. I mean it brings this message of self-care home to me in a much different way.

Marcia: Yeah. You know what? I don't want people to wait until the end of their lives to know that their lives mattered. That's really my heartfelt deep message to everyone listening and to myself. Let's practice today seeing what's meaningful and what's precious about our life, our loves and our relationships. Let's take a moment in gratitude and in appreciation and let's have the courage to say no more and no thank you to the things that are sucking the life out of us that we're complaining about that are no longer in integrity with our soul. As we say no more to what's no longer true, we can say now what to truly that which is meaningful and to that which really does matter to us. That's what a well-lived life every moment of every day and every day of our lives I think is really all about.

Kevin: Beautiful.

Harmony: I just want to thank you, Marcia, for your vulnerability and your truth telling. It's obvious to me that you're a leader of a lot of people and that you lead by your experience. By you talking about really looking for the meaning of meaning in your life, it's obvious to me that you're really going for the depth and I thank you for sharing your vulnerability with us.

Marcia: Well, that means so much to me. I really appreciate that reflection. It is true that this upcoming event of the Wealthy Visionary Conference will be highly experiential and every single thing that I teach is something I've lived through. I have a funny new little saying, you guys will appreciate it. Been to hell, lived to tell about it, must be here to teach about it. Each of us have lived through our stories and those of us that are visionaries, certainly all of us listening in and participating in the Self-Care Revolution™, we do have big dreams. We do have our good days and our bad days and I think when we're willing to just authentically say I'm struggling, I don't know, I'm figuring it out or I lived through this challenging thing, here's what I learned and maybe it can be useful for you, then I think we truly are sharing our gifts and at one level what's more meaningful than that.

Robyn: Yes. I know in our very first interview with you, you shared more of your story, some of your hell in your life. For all of you that are listening just know that every single interview we've done is in a wonderful book. We're going to have the whole 12-month series, all the modules available to each and every one of you. Again, rich content, lots of deep meaning that's been shared throughout these 12 months.

So, Marcia, we have the time for one more question. As you go into your next year, maybe talk about your self-care rituals. I just saw you speak at the Rituals Conference and the importance of rituals, maybe share a little bit about that in terms of how that brings meaning into life and what your self-care lifestyle looks like.

Marcia: Sure. I want to just say I saw the book just from the first month and the level of richness and content. I think the fact that you've put it together and made this available where people can listen to the program, read the transcripts and really have the book and the materials on their shelf. I do have it correct; they can actually get a hard copy of it?

Robyn: Exactly.

Marcia: For me, that book becomes part of my library and part of my self-care is to have that kind of reference material available. Sometimes I use it as a tool of Divination. I'll just go to the shelf and I'll reach for what feels true. I could open up this book on self-care and any passage from any one of the extraordinary speakers is going to offer me wisdom, insight and gifts. There are so many tools, but then it's the remembering to use them, so I think I'm going to continue in this practice of being highly focused.

My company used to put on seven events a year. Now we're only putting on the Wealthy Visionary Conference, one big, substantial, in-depth event. So that's a focusing tool for me. This year I set the intention to go on two fabulous exotic vacations to places I hadn't been to. I went to Marrakech and to the Galapagos Islands and I found I'm just so happy when I'm exploring something that new. I reminded myself that I don't have to fly to the other side of the world and that there are places in L.A. I've never even been to.

One thing is to get really clear about what brings me joy and spend more time doing what makes me joyful, so the exploration. I've made meeting my beloved and my soul mate my highest priority for 2014, so really looking at what are the things that I, personally, need and want to do to make that happen. On a simple level, it's really taking care of my body and nurturing my heart and soul so I feel beautiful and I have energy and my light is fully turned on and illuminated. On a practical sense, it's asking for what I need, having friends fix me up and doing some online dating. Even sharing it here and now it's very vulnerable for me to put out to the world that what I want more than anything is to be in love with my beloved and my soul mate and just spending more time with people that I love.

I have a lot of people in my life, but I really want more circles of conscious people, so joining my temple or going to the Kabala centers. For me, it's always this mixture of the inner and the outer, so what are the inner practices and rituals, the inner of really feeling what I need, the inner of when I'm hungry reaching for something healthy and nurturing, whatever is going to make me happy in that moment, the inner of my prayer and my meditation time and laying on my mat that you got me, so doing the right things on a regular basis.

Mostly I could sum it up by where we started and that is the ongoing practice of everyday enlightenment. Not just what I'm thinking and saying, but what I'm doing and who I'm doing it with and really at the end of the day tying it all up with this bow of seeking, finding and doing more of what is meaningful for me and really acknowledging and appreciating it. I think that that really is my prescription.

My Grandma Fritzy who dies in her 80's used to say nothing ages you faster than stinkin' thinkin'. When I think about Grandma Fritzy she said to me, just live every day so if you close your eyes when you go to sleep and you don't wake up you can die happy and fulfilled. I practiced that a lot when I was younger and then I got busy. I got consumed by work and worry and money and other kinds of issues and stuff and this is my time to return to that practice of really living every day and helping every day to be meaningful and fulfilling so that whatever life has in store for me I'm able to really meet it in a way that is precious and perfect.

Robyn: Woo-hoo!

Marcia: Thank you for asking, such a really good question. You guys always ask such good questions. I've got to just tell you, I'm so honored. Ritual has a beginning, middle and end and for me, personally, the fact that I kicked off your series. I was your very first speaker and I'm ending your series as your very last speaker, for me, it's just a reminder that this whole experience has been a ritual. I know it's a ritual that transformed your lives by conceiving it, creating it and fulfilling upon the dream and the promise, but as one of your speakers I wanted to bring in that it's such a ritual.

It's been a very rewarding ritual for me to participate and to really be here at the end to punctuate the experience and to really acknowledge and appreciate you for what you've created. All of the thousands and thousands of lives and then the ripple effect, the tens of hundreds of thousands of lives, all the way to your goal of a billion, that will be awakened through this ritual of what we've created. I was a contributor, but what we've all created and how holy it's been. You created something incredibly meaningful, incredibly important and incredibly valuable and on behalf of all of the speakers that have participated, allow me to bow my head in deep gratitude and appreciation for what you've created and the impact that it not only has had, but will continue to have in the years and years to come.

Robyn: Oh, thank you so much. You are a blessing. We wish you the most fabulous New Year and we can't wait to read your meaningful book. Again, thank you for the profound meaning you've brought to this Revolution and saying yes to start with you and your message and to end. We can't wait to see you live in just a few months.

Marcia: I know! I'm so excited. We'll see you at the Wealthy Visionary Conference. Please come join us. Kevin, thank you.

Kevin: Absolutely. Thank you. Thank you for taking us from dreaming to meaning.

Robyn: Whoa! What a way to bookend the year. We love you. You take care and we look forward to seeing you soon. Lots of love.

Marcia: Thanks. Bye to you, too, Harmony. Much love, blessings.

Harmony: Thank you, too, Marcia, bye.

Marcia: Bye-bye.

[End of Interview]

www.ingramcontent.com/pod-product-compliance
Lightning Source LLC
Chambersburg PA
CBHW080414290526
45791CB00008BA/2273